A GUIDE TO MEDICAL CARE ADMINISTRATION

Volume II

**MEDICAL CARE APPRAISAL—
QUALITY AND UTILIZATION**

The American Public Health Association
1015 Eighteenth Street N.W.
Washington, D.C. 200036

COPYRIGHT 1969 BY THE AMERICAN PUBLIC HEALTH ASSOCIATION, INC.
Library of Congress Catalog No. 65–26944
SBN NUMBER: 87553–012–5

Fourth Printing 1975

A GUIDE TO MEDICAL CARE ADMINISTRATION

Volume II:

MEDICAL CARE APPRAISAL— QUALITY AND UTILIZATION

Prepared By
AVEDIS DONABEDIAN, M.D.

As an activity of
The Program Area Committee on Medical Care Administration
of the American Public Health Association
in cooperation with the Division of Medical Care Administration
of the U.S. Public Health Service.
Supported by Public Health Service Contract PH 108–66–153.

Program Area Committee on
Medical Care Administration—1965–1968
of the
American Public Health Association

1965–1968	CECIL G. SHEPS, M.D. *(Chairman)*
	JOHN W. CASHMAN, M.D.
	NORMAN R. INGRAHAM, JR., M.D.
	LEONARD ROSENFELD, M.D.
	E. RICHARD WEINERMAN, M.D.
1965–1967	MADELYN HALL, R.N.
1965–1966	BERNARD BUCOVE, M.D.
	F. BURNS ROTH, M.D.
	QUENTIN M. SMITH, D.D.S.
1966–1967	LESTER BRESLOW, M.D.
1966–1968	JEROME POLLACK, ED.D.
	SELVIN SONKEN, D.D.S.
1967–1968	ROBERT WHALEN, M.D.

Staff to the Committee

1966–1967	BEVERLEE A. MYERS, M.P.H.
1967–1968	A. GERALD RENTHAL, M.D.

Participants
Workshop on Medical Care Appraisal—Operational Aspects
November 11–12, 1966

Speakers

MIKELBANK, G.
"Approval by Individual Diagnosis (AID) Program of New Jersey Blue Cross"

Director
Department of Hospital Utilization
Hospital Services Plan of New Jersey

MOREHEAD, MILDRED A., M.D.
"The Medical Audit as an Operational Tool"

Associate Professor of Administrative Medicine
Columbia University School of Public Health

PAYNE, BEVERLY C., M.D.
"A Criteria Approach to Measurement of Quality of Medical Care and Effectiveness of Use of the Hospital"

Assistant Dean
University of Michigan
School of Medicine

SCHAEFFER, MORRIS, M.D.
"An Appraisal of the Clinical Laboratories in New York City"

Director
Bureau of Laboratories
New York City Department of Health

SHAPIRO, SAM
"End Result Measurement of Quality of Medical Care"

Director
Division of Research and Statistics
Health Insurance Plan of Greater New York

SHINDELL, SIDNEY, M.D.
"Hospital Utilization Review—Western Pennsylvania"

Head
Department of Preventive Medicine
Marquette University

SLEE, VERGIL, M.D.
"CPHA Experience in Measuring Quality"

Director
Commission on Professional Activities

Discussants

DENSEN, PAUL D.SC.
Papers by Payne and Slee

Deputy Administrator
Health Services Administration
City of New York

RIEDEL, DONALD C., PH.D.
Papers by Mikelbank and Shindell

Associate Professor of Public Health
Yale University School of Medicine

SHEPS, MINDEL C., M.D.
Papers by Morehead, Schaeffer and Shapiro

Professor of Biostatistics
Columbia University
School of Public Health

PARTICIPANTS

Invited Guests

BREWSTER, AGNES
Bureau of State Services
Medical Care Administration
Public Health Service

SONKEN, SELVIN, D.D.S.
Chief
Dental Care Administration
Bureau of State Services
Public Health Service

MYERS, BEVERLEE A., M.P.H.
Deputy Chief
Health Services Organization Branch
Division of Medical Care Administration
Public Health Service

RICHARDSON, FRED, M.D.
Acting Project Director
Research and Medical Review Methodology
Albany

American Public Health Association

HOOD, THOMAS R., M.D.
Deputy Executive Director
American Public Health Association

Program Area Committee on Medical Care Administration

SHEPS, CECIL G., M.D. *(Chairman)*
General Director
Beth Israel Medical Center

INGRAHAM, NORMAN R., M.D.
Health Commissioner
Philadelphia Department of Health

ROSENFELD, LEONARD, M.D.
Director
Division of Medical Services
Hospital Review and Planning Council of Southern New York

ROTH, F. BURNS, M.D.
Chairman
Department of Health Administration
University of Toronto
School of Hygiene

SMITH, QUENTIN M., D.D.S.
Regional Dental Consultant
Department of Health, Education and Welfare
Regional Office
Atlanta

WEINERMAN, E. RICHARD, M.D.
Professor of Medicine and Public Health
Yale University School of Medicine

Table of Contents

Author-Editor's Preface ix
Foreword and Acknowledgments xi

Part I:

FRAME OF REFERENCE 1
    Approaches to Appraisal 2
    Levels of Concern 5
    Definition of Quality 7
    Further Development of Material 13

Part II:

SELECTED METHODS OF APPRAISAL 14
Summary of Classification of Methods 14
Appraisal of Process 14
    Certification 14
    Statistical Display and Analysis 21
    Case Review 27
    Appraisal of the Data Used for Clinical Decision Making .. 28
Appraisal of End Results 31

Part III:

ISSUES OF METHOD AND TECHNIQUE 42
    Some General Requirements 42
    Sources of Information 42
    Sampling and Selection 52
    Standards 62
    Measurement Scales 77
    Reliability, Validity and Bias 81
    Indices of Medical Care 93
    Integrative Appraisal of Quality 96

TABLE OF CONTENTS

Part IV:

ISSUES OF POLICY AND IMPLEMENATION 99
   Objectives of Appraisal 99
   Responsibility for Appraisal 104
   Implementation 116
   Costs 121
   Effectiveness 122
   Dangers 151

Part V:

FURTHER RESEARCH AND DEVELOPMENT 153

Part VI:

SYNTHESIS AND CONCLUSIONS 160

REFERENCES 166
ANNOTATED SELECTED BIBLIOGRAPHY 177
   Description and Evaluation of Methods of Appraisal 179
   Research Studies and Applications: Methods and Findings.. 188
   Implementation and Effectiveness of Utilization Review ... 213
   Standards 217
   Evaluation in Nursing 219
   Drug Therapy Audit 221

Author-Editor's Preface

This volume of the *Guide to Medical Care Administration* began with two sources of basic materials: (1) a set of seven papers prepared at the request of the Program Area Committee on Medical Care Administration and (2) a stenotyped transcript of the proceedings of a workshop during which these papers were presented and discussed. More specifically, the workshop transcript offered three kinds of material: (1) verbal presentations by the authors of the papers, (2) a critique of each paper by a designated discussant, and (3) general discussion, in the course of which authors replied to questions and criticism. A list of authors (with the titles of their papers), discussants and other workshop participants is given beginning on pages v and vi.

The task of preparing Volume II of the Guide was originally conceived to consist of editing and pulling together the basic materials mentioned. It soon became clear, however, that the scope of the volume had to be enlarged to round out information in the basic materials and to incorporate additional, and sometimes more recent, information. The volume has therefore grown beyond original expectations. As it now stands, it is perhaps the most exhaustive discussion of the theoretical and operational aspects of medical care appraisal currently available.

In preparing this volume, the author-editor has recast the material in the basic sources with which he started, and additional materials from the literature on appraisal, into a rather personal framework of concepts and categories. To do this he has had to make extensive use of his own previous publications and of unpublished materials he developed for use in his teaching. The resultant framework of concepts and categories was used to prepare an extensive classification of issues pertaining to appraisal. A card index of abstracts was then prepared of all the relevant items in the seven basic papers and the workshop transcript. This method gives considerable assurance that although the material has been reshaped into a more general form, no significant items of information in the basic materials have been lost. Moreover, because meticulous attention was given to recording the sources of information, it is hoped that in all instances authorship and verbal contributions have been appropriately recognized.

The usefulness of this volume is believed to be greatly enhanced by the Annotated Bibliography so ably assembled and abstracted by Miss Alice Anderson. The papers cited were selected with special emphasis on (1) utilization; (2) on "the process of medical care and end results" [defined herein]; (3) on methodology in general, or (4) on the ap-

PREFACE

plication of a given method. Items relating to nursing care, drug therapy, and standards are presented to indicate some representative studies, but are by no means intended to cover these areas comprehensively. Studies in mental health have been omitted entirely, this area calling for an extensive bibliography in itself. Evaluations of community programs, such as screening or immunization programs, have not been cited, with one or two exceptions. Likewise, no effort was made to annotate reports on medical care in any country other than the United States. The classification used to group the abstracts was devised to achieve the greatest possible congruence with the arrangement of the material and the terminology used in the text.

In conclusion, it is a pleasure to acknowledge help and encouragement received from many sources. First, the author-editor recognizes his indebtedness to the Program Area Committee on Medical Care Administration for asking him to prepare this volume and for making available the excellent source materials that form its nucleus. He is also indebted to the agencies that have supported and published his previous work on quality appraisal, which material has been drawn upon freely in the preparation of this volume (see references 1, 5, 26, 58, 154, 155 and 158).

Mr. Jack Tobias, librarian to the Reference Collection in Medical Care Administration at the University of Michigan, has, as always, rendered valuable bibliographic help. The manuscript, exclusive of the Annotated Bibliography, was typed by Mrs. Sarah Giancola, who also managed all those aspects of production which took place in Ann Arbor. Without her able participation this volume could not have met the deadline set for its completion.

Perhaps most important of all, credit is due to the School of Public Health at the University of Michigan and, in particular, to its Department of Medical Care Organization, for creating and assiduously nurturing the academic environment within which the author-editor has been able to pursue, with a minimum of distraction, his scholarly interests and his teaching.

Ann Arbor
August 21, 1968

AVEDIS DONABEDIAN, M.D.

Foreword And Acknowledgments

This is the second volume in a series that was developed by the Program Area Committee on Medical Care Administration of the American Public Health Association. The first was originally published in 1965 and was entitled *Concepts and Principles*. It was widely used and is being reprinted, with modest revisions, in conjunction with the publication of this volume.

In addition to a series of discussions at meetings of the Program Area Committee, Volume II is based, in large measure, upon a workshop on the operational aspects of medical care appraisal which was held on November 11 and 12, 1966. The plans for this workshop were developed by a subcommittee consisting of Drs. L. S. Rosenfeld, E. R. Weinerman and C. G. Sheps.

The Program Area Committee is deeply indebted to Dr. Avedis Donabedian, who took on the responsibility of being the author-editor. He has not only functioned as an editor, but has rounded out and greatly improved upon the workshop materials by adding new materials and bringing in his own concepts.

This volume has been supplemented by an annotated bibliography which was prepared by Miss Alice Anderson. Relevant details regarding the purpose, organization and preparation of the book are outlined in the author-editor's preface.

Major credit for guiding the transition of this work from manuscript form to publication belongs to Miss Margaret Pierce, Assistant Publications Editor of the American Public Health Association and to Dr. Gerald Renthal, Staff to the Program Area Committee on Medical Care Administration.

This publication provides a theoretical and operational discussion of selected methods of appraising the quality of medical care. Major attention is given to the appraisal of the *process* of medical care and the *assessment of outcomes*. As the text states, ". . . this volume is concerned with methods that can keep the quality of care under constant surveillance." It is hoped that it will be useful to those who have administrative responsibility, responsibility for clinical performance and also to those who are interested in further research. The text, references and the annotated bibliography should be widely useful.

> CECIL G. SHEPS, M.D., *Chairman*
> Program Area Committee on Medical Care Administration
> American Public Health Association

April, 1969

Part I:

FRAME OF REFERENCE

The present volume deals with the appraisal of medical care. It does so within a fairly specific framework, which this section attempts to define.

First of all, this is a guide for the administrator. Accordingly, the emphasis is on assuring the quality of medical care in operating programs. The approach, however, is not operational in the sense that the administrator is given rules of thumb for what to do and what not to do. Administrative action is the objective; but this is mediated by developing a sensitive understanding of the basic issues and factors in the appraisal of medical care. The administrator is then equipped to evaluate the methods now at hand, to adapt them to his purposes, and to participate in the further development and evaluation of new methods as they emerge.

Although this volume deals with methods of appraisal as a means to assuring the quality of medical care, the reader must remember that the basic safeguard of the quality of care is appropriate program design. A proper design must take into account the nature and scope of program benefits, the conditions under which clients may participate, the standards governing the participation and the professional practice of the providers of care, methods of financing, and methods and terms of payment. It also includes the mobilization and proper organization of the resources, human and other, that are needed for the delivery of care. Mechanisms for the appraisal of care are but one, though essential, element in the overall design. They are essential because they alone provide tangible proof that the system operates as it should and, where it does not, they indicate areas that need attention and improvement. Program design must, therefore, be constantly subject to the test of performance.

In medical care settings with any degree of organization there are a number of formal and informal activities which involve explicit or implicit judgments on the quality of care rendered. Examples of these activities would include clinical and clinical-pathological conferences, patient rounds, referrals and consultations, as well as exchanges with junior colleagues and students in the course of teaching and training. All these interactions are credited with exerting a powerful influence on performance—deriving partly from the spirit of inquiry, said to be fostered by such activities, which is conducive to constant learning, and partly because the very visibility of care

STRUCTURE

to colleagues competent to judge it is an incentive to maintain standards.

The scope of this volume does not embrace all activities of formal or informal appraisal but is limited to a small number of formally instituted mechanisms designed to exert a fairly specific control function—although the control function may not be the exclusive, or even major, purpose.

The administrative frame of reference would appear to impose still another restriction on the scope of this volume, namely the exclusion of research objectives and orientations. This is only partly true. The emphasis in this volume is indeed on those methods of appraisal that can monitor, constantly or repeatedly, the quality of care for which a program has assumed responsibility. But the monitoring methods, or variants of them, can also be used to study the consequences of planned change or to compare one form of organization with another preparatory to making a choice between them. As such they become tools for operational research and evaluation. Furthermore, insightful examination of the quality of care, as revealed by these methods, can raise significant questions that should initiate further research, basic and applied. The administrative appraisal of the quality of care is, therefore, seen to merge into the research use of identical or similar methods; and administrative appraisal constitutes one end of a continuum that is linked, through the medium of operational research, with more traditional research activities.

Approaches to Appraisal

Three major approaches to the evaluation of quality have been identified. These have been designated as the evaluation of *structure, process,* and *outcome* or end results.[1]

Appraisal of structure involves the evaluation of the settings and instrumentalities available and used for the provision of care. While including the physical aspects of facilities and equipment, structural appraisal goes far beyond to encompass the characteristics of the administrative organization and the qualifications of health professionals. The term *structure,* as used here, also signifies the properties of the resources used to provide care and the manner in which they are organized.

Two major assumptions are made when structure is taken as an indicator of quality: First, that better care is more likely to be provided when better qualified staff, improved physical facilities and sounder fiscal and administrative organization are employed. Second, that we know enough to identify what is "good" in terms of staff, physical structure and formal organization. That staff qualifications, physical structure and formal organization are not equated with quality must be emphasized. It is only expected that there is a relationship between these structural elements and the quality of care, so that, given good structural properties, good care is more likely (though not certain) to occur. Devices like licensure, certification of facilities, and accreditation are based largely on this assumption.

Assessment of process is the evaluation of the activities of physicians and other health professionals in the management of patients. The criterion generally used is the degree to which management of patients conforms with the standards and expectations of the respective professions. These standards and expectations may be derived from what is considered to be "ideal," "good," or "acceptable" practice as formulated by recognized leaders in the profession. Such standards may also be inferred from patterns of care observed in actual practice. One or more institutions or groups of professionals that are expected to give good care may be taken as the standard, and other providers compared to this standard. Alternatively, institutions or health professionals can be compared with each other in order to try to establish averages and ranges in health care activities. Interpretation of the observed patterns rests on professional judgment with or without further study of the factors related to the occurrence of unusual patterns of care.

When evaluation of process is the basis for judgments concerning quality, a major assumption is that health care is useful in maintaining or promoting health. Furthermore, there is the explicit or implicit assumption that particular elements and aspects of care are known to be specifically related to successful or unsuccessful health outcomes or end results.

Assessment of outcomes is the evaluation of end results in terms of health and satisfaction. That this evaluation in many ways provides the final evidence of whether care has been good, bad or indifferent is so because of the broad fundamental social and professional agreement on what results are deemed desirable. Furthermore, it is assumed that good results are brought about, at least to a significant degree, by good care.

It is generally conceded that the appraisal of structure is too indirect to be definitive. Beyond this, there tends to be a curious polarization of opinion concerning the relative merits of the assessment of process and of outcome, a polarization which arises, not so much from technical considerations, as from different concepts of what constitute the terms of reference and the objectives of administrative appraisal. Those who focus on process point out that their responsibility is to see to it that "the best" medical care, as defined by health experts, is provided. They do not consider it their primary concern to evaluate the effectiveness of the health sciences. By contrast, those who would focus on outcomes or end results emphasize primary concern for health and for the responsibility of the administrator to investigate the causes of failure to achieve health objectives and to take appropriate action.

This volume will espouse the viewpoint that the identification of three approaches to appraisal does not mean that they are independent of each other or that one has to be selected in preference to the other. On the contrary, it should now be clear that the three approaches are interrelated. Appropriate structure increases the probability of good care, which, in turn, improves the likelihood of favorable outcomes. It is recognized that the precise interrelationships are not fully understood and that there is need for much further research to elucidate fully the relationships between structure and process, process and outcome, and structure and outcome. It is also recognized that, pending the development of further knowledge, quality can be assessed by all three approaches using what is currently known or believed about these interrelationships. The three approaches are, in fact, mutually reinforcing; and any operational system of appraisal should probably incorporate elements of all three. The total information obtained when all three approaches are used simultaneously may well be greater than the mere sum of the three, since knowledge of the interrelations among them gives a deeper understanding of the state of the patient's care.

As stated, the present volume is concerned with methods that can keep the quality of care under constant surveillance. Since structural elements are relatively fixed, and are slow to change, the emphasis in this volume will be on selected methods for the appraisal of process and of end results. This does not mean that under certain circumstances the evaluation of structural features may not be the procedure of choice or one important element additional to the evaluation of process and of end results. Most standards of program design and operation promulgated by professional associations and governmental agencies rest on the specification of structural features. Goldmann [142] and Weinerman,[143] among others, have demonstrated the usefulness of structural analysis in program evaluation. Such evaluations, however, are not considered to be primarily tools for continuous surveillance. It is for this reason that they have been excluded from the present volume. The reader should note this important exclusion from Volume II and judge its relevance to his own needs accordingly.

Levels of Concern

Another aspect of the framework within which appraisal of the quality of care is to be carried out is specification of the level and scope of administrative concern. The way in which these are defined is determined partly by the mission of the agency that engages in appraisal, and partly by technical and other considerations that determine which approach to appraisal is most feasible.

Concern may encompass the overall health of an entire population or a specified subgroup of a larger population. For example, this is the appropriate frame of reference for planning at the national, state, or local levels. It is also appropriate, and necessary, for discharging the mission of a prepaid group practice which assumes responsibility for providing "comprehensive" care for its enrollees.

In other situations, concern may be limited to the quality of care which an agency itself provides. A hospital, a clinic, or an individual physician may strive to provide the best care possible to patients, without assuming guardianship for the health of an entire population. Yet this is valid because the mission of these providers is more narrowly defined.

There is an intermediate level of concern. Providers, while not assuming responsibility for the health of a definable population, may accept responsibility for the entire care of clients, even though care is received from a multiplicity of sources. Such responsibility would be not only appropriate but also essential on the part of any provider that functions as a "central source of care" for any given client.[2-4]

As already indicated, the defined level of concern has important implications for quality appraisal. Assumption of responsibility for the health of an entire population requires that the population in question be clearly definable. For example, the inability to define clearly its population base may be a significant contributory factor limiting the ability of a hospital to expand its concern beyond the care it provides to clients. Concern for an entire population, or for the entire care received by a group of clients, requires evaluation of the care received from several sources and given by many types of professional and other providers. Such evaluation encounters severe problems of access to information. Furthermore, techniques for assessing the care provided by professional personnel other than physicians and nurses are still rudimentary. Even were it possible to evaluate successfully the quality of care offered by each provider involved in the care of a given client, there would remain problems of assessing the manner in which these different components are fitted together to achieve health objectives. Because of these difficulties, assessment of outcomes, rather than of process, is the approach generally used when the level of concern embraces entire populations or the totality of care. Evaluation of process is generally reserved for those situations in which concern is for the care directly under the control of the provider. This does not mean that outcomes cannot be also used to assess care at this more proximate level of concern. There is, however, an affinity between all-embracing responsibilities and the use of similarly all-embracing measures of health and well-being. When the concerns are more sharply focused on particular episodes of care, the indicators of outcome are more precisely chosen to relate to these particular episodes.

Another aspect of assessment that is keyed closely to the level of concern is the degree of emphasis on access to care as a dimension of quality. When the concern embraces an entire population, it is usual to place great emphasis on access or lack of access to care as a major indicator of quality in the system. It avails the population little if a minority that has ready access to care receives excellent care when large numbers are denied access or are seriously handicapped in obtaining adequate care. When the level of concern is more narrowly defined, access is a matter of lesser saliency since attention is focused on the quality of care delivered by providers to clients who have already gained access to care. Even within this narrower framework, access to care can be a sensitive indicator of provider performance. This is because access to care is influenced both directly and indirectly by provider actions and the nature of the provider-client interaction, currently and in the past. The provider is certainly instrumental in routing the client through the various units that comprise the medical care system. Past experience with care is likely to be a significant factor in determining whether care is sought or avoided, just as current experience can determine the degree of compliance with physician recommendations. These arguments notwithstanding, access to care may receive less attention than it deserves in the assessment of provider performance, for one or more of the following reasons: the influence of the provider on initial access to care is considered to be small; the individual provider, or the providers collectively, are considered not to have social responsibility for assuring access to care; the provider's responsibility for access, though significant, is considered to rank lower in the order of priorities of concern than other provider actions of greater moment; or it is difficult to obtain and evaluate relevant information.[5]

The degree of emphasis on access is one aspect of a more general issue that is germane to the level of concern, namely proper allocation of health resources. At the population level, concern is with the distribution of health services in a manner that assures the best health possible for all. In actual practice, this may necessitate lowering the quality of care for certain groups of the population in order to raise the average quality of care, and health levels, for all.

It is clear, therefore, that a definition of the level of concern is an essential prelude to the choice of indicators of quality and to the institution of appropriate methods of appraisal.

In this volume the frame of reference is defined rather narrowly so as to permit concentration on evaluation of the care furnished the clients of an agency that provides or purchases care. Furthermore, concern is almost exclusively with the care provided by physicians, which is not to say that care provided by other professionals is not worthy of similar attention. It does, however, indicate that the greatest amount of work has so far been done in the evaluation of physician care. Hence, this represents the most highly developed area of knowledge in methods of appraisal. Fortunately, many of the methodological and policy issues pertaining to the evaluation of physician care should also be relevant to assessment of the care provided by other health professionals, and to that extent this volume should have applicability beyond assessment of the services of physicians.

Definition of Quality

A final element in the framework that shapes and supports any system of quality appraisal is the definition of quality upon which that system rests. The quality of medical care is extraordinarily difficult to define because one must first indicate what dimensions or aspects of care are subject to consideration and then specify what constitutes "goodness" or "badness" with respect to these aspects or dimensions.

The specification of relevant dimensions is a matter of considerable difficulty because medical care comprises a complex set of interactions. These include provider behaviors, client behaviors and client-provider interactions. Each of these behaviors or interactions is further subdivided into many elements and related to a host of organizational and social factors that play upon it.

Even more difficult is specifying what "goodness" is. Judgment of what is good derives from the standards of management acceptable to leaders of the profession at any given time. Since these standards apply to particular situations, they must be specified in almost endless detail. Moreover, the standards reflect current knowledge and orientations, and are subject to change as knowledge advances and the scope of provider responsibility is redefined. The definition of provider responsibility is itself only partly a matter of professional determination. It is arrived at by a social process in which the profession participates in conjunction with others.[5]

DEFINITION OF QUALITY

These difficulties notwithstanding, it is possible to offer at least partial definitions of quality that identify certain properties of provider performance, of the provider-client relationship, and of outcomes which either signify "goodness" or need to be taken into account in making a judgment about quality. Some examples will illustrate the utility and limitations of these partial definitions.

Payne has defined quality as "that level of excellence produced and documented in the process of diagnosis and therapy, based on the best knowledge derived from science and the humanities, and which eventuates in the least morbidity and mortality in the population."[6] Esselstyn offers the following definition: "Standards of quality of care should be based on the degree to which care is available, acceptable, comprehensive, continuous, and documented, as well as on the extent to which adequate therapy is based on accurate diagnosis and not on symptomatology."[7]

Lee and Jones in their classic work, *The Fundamentals of Good Medical Care*,[8] define quality as follows: "Good medical care is the kind of medicine practiced and taught by the recognized leaders of the medical profession at a given time or period of social, cultural, and professional development in a community or population group. ... The concept of good medical care that has been employed in this study is based upon certain 'articles of faith' which can be briefly stated.

1. Good medical care is limited to the practice of rational medicine based on the medical sciences.
2. Good medical care emphasizes prevention.
3. Good medical care requires intelligent cooperation between the lay public and the practitioners of scientific medicine.
4. Good medical care treats the individual as a whole.
5. Good medical care maintains a close and continuing personal relation between physician and patient.
6. Good medical care is coordinated with social welfare work.
7. Good medical care coordinates all types of medical services.
8. Good medical care implies the application of all the necessary services of modern scientific medicine to the needs of all the people."

More recently, Donabedian has expanded the Lee-Jones "articles" into a more detailed listing of relevant aspects of physician behavior and the client-physician relationship (Reference 5, Appendix A).

None of the definitions cited constitutes a determination of goodness in any particular situation. However, they do identify what might be called dimensions of quality and assert that a statement concerning quality in any particular situation is not complete unless judgments are made concerning each of these dimensions. For example, Article 2 of the Lee-Jones definition makes the point that the degree to which management fully exploits opportunities for preventive intervention needs to be determined and evaluated. What, precisely, those opportunities are depends on the situation and on what medical science has to offer for that situation; and on whether the full application of preventive measures is advisable in the light of competing priorities.

It may be indicative of a pervasive bias in conceptualizing quality, and in approaches to its assessment, that almost all the dimensions identified as relevant to quality pertain to process rather than outcome. Payne's definition is the exception, in indicating a necessary relationship between process and outcome. Furthermore, the definitions cited show central concern with the management of patients. The Payne definition is exclusively occupied with the technical aspects of care; the other two add considerations of the patient-physician relationship. It is also interesting that both Payne and Esselstyn emphasize recording as a dimension of quality in the management of patients.

Although the major preoccupation, in these definitions, appears to be with management of patients, there are indications of broader concern. Esselstyn considers "availability" a dimension of quality. Article 8 of the Lee-Jones definition deserves special attention because it transcends the care of a particular client by a particular provider, dealing with the manner in which the total capabilities of the medical care system are deployed in the interests of all the people, including those who do not receive service even though they need it.

The definitions cited also illustrate clearly the notion that assessment of quality involves judgments of "goodness" applied to many components and attributes of the medical care process. Comprehensive assessment would obviously be difficult. It is more usual for appraisal to focus on a few facts or aspects and neglect many others. In particular, most assessments focus on the more traditional facets of technical professional performance. Often excluded are certain elements of technical performance, such as prevention and rehabilitation. Even more frequently excluded are considerations of the social and psychological management of illness and health, integration of the management of illness and health, coordination and continuity of care, aspects of the client-provider relationship (covering also client and provider satisfaction), and considerations of economic efficiency or the optimum allocation of resources. An important task, then, is to determine how inclusive the definition of quality is to be.

Another problem is that direct or indirect participants in the medical care process and the provision of health services are likely to conceive differently the relative importance of the various components of care and the criteria of "goodness" with respect to each. Hence, clients, providers, administrators, planners and economists may differ

DEFINITION OF QUALITY

significantly in their views of quality. Especially significant to any definitions would be disparate views between physicians and patients and between administrators and physicians as to what constitutes quality. Disparities of opinion between patients and physicians may account, in part, for the continued popularity of incompetent, or comparatively less competent, health practitioners.

A third problem arising out of the multipartite nature of quality is that of determining the degree to which there are internal conflicts or incompatibilities among the various components. This implies that the achievement of quality in one component of care may be associated with a tendency to deterioration in another. Is it possible, for example, that technical excellence may tend to be associated with fragmentation and impersonality of care? If this were true, special attention might need to be directed, in the process of appraisal, to those dimensions of quality that appear to be in conflict. Such possibilities also have important implications for the organization of service. Services ought to be organized so as to minimize such conflicts. In some situations it may be difficult to achieve comparable levels of excellence in all components of care. Priorities may need to be set up and difficult choices may have to be made.

Another critical question concerns the performance of the individual practitioner, or a given institution. Is performance homogeneous with respect to the many components of care? How likely is it that a physician who performs well or badly in diagnosing illness will perform similarly in treatment, or in the management of the patient-physician relationship? Furthermore, is a physician's performance uniform across the range of health and illness with which he customarily deals, or does it differ significantly from one disease category to another? Is care in one department of a hospital provided at a level of quality comparable to that provided in another department of the same hospital? The answers to these questions have important implications for the way in which care must be assessed. If levels of performance are essentially uniform for an individual provider or within an institution, the task of quality assessment is considerably simplified. It is possible to select a few situations and a small number of care components to represent the overall performance of each provider. It will also be possible to characterize the performance of each practitioner as good, bad or indifferent. Where performance is not uniform or homogeneous, careful sampling becomes a critical element in methods of assessment. It may be impossible to characterize performance by a single adjective; rather, one may have to evaluate performance separately with respect to each component of care, and to construct a "profile" for each provider.[9]

There will be further discussion of the issues of multidimensionality and heterogeneity of care in subsequent sections of this volume. In addition, the rather meager empirical findings will be summarized. At this point it is only necessary to introduce the concept that quality may not be a simple attribute of a unidimensional phenomenon. The probable complexity of the situation is empirically illustrated in a study by Klein *et al.*, who found that 24 "administrative officials" gave 80 different criteria for evaluating patient care. The authors concluded that patient care, like morale, cannot be considered a unitary concept and that ". . . it seems likely there will never be a single comprehensive criterion by which to measure the quality of care."[10]

Fortunately, there are a number of factors that tend to unify medical care and to simplify its appraisal. For one, an integrative process within the individual practitioner may result in close correspondence of performance in the different aspects of care. Through a variety of organizational mechanisms a similar, though less complete, homogeneity may characterize the performance of a medical institution. In fact, there may be a measurable "overall capacity for goodness in medical care" as postulated by Peterson and his coworkers.[11] Moreover, one can count on a certain all-or-none property to medical care which, if it fails seriously in any one critical component, can be said to have failed as a whole. This may make it possible to characterize the quality of a sequence of care by the properties of the weakest critical link.

Significant to the definition of quality is the relationship between quantity and quality, hence between the appraisal of quality and of utilization. It is a truism that quantity is a necessary precondition to quality. Attention does not begin to center on quality unless the most urgent considerations of minimum care have already been met. The absence of necessary or appropriate care connotes the absence of quality. Deficiencies due to omissions are just as significant as those that arise out of commissions—and deserve equal attention in appraisal. These remarks are especially germane to utilization review, which currently seems to place preponderant emphasis on excessive use without enough concern for insufficient use. Concern for length of stay, for example, is expressed almost entirely in terms of overstay, with little attention to inappropriately short stays. In this connection, a study of Michigan hospitals has shown that, for a specified list of common diagnoses, inappropriately short stays, though fewer than inappropriately long stays, are by no means negligible. In this study, inappropriately long stays accounted for 9.6 percent of hospital discharges and 6.8 percent of patient days, whereas inappropriately short stays accounted for 6.8 percent of discharges and 2.3 percent of patient days. Among those patients who bore the entire cost of medical care,

DEFINITION OF QUALITY

inappropriately short stays were more frequent than inappropriately long stays.[12]

Excessive use is also justifiably interpreted as poor quality, and for several reasons. Procedures performed may be inappropriate and potentially harmful, even though actual harm to the patient may occur infrequently. This is certainly true for unnecessary surgery, since any surgery always carries some risk, no matter how small. It is also true for unnecessary hospitalization, since all hospitalization implies some risk of hospital-acquired infection, atrophy of disuse and trauma, as well as social and psychological damage. These dangers, especially of atrophy of disuse or social and psychological damage, are magnified when hospitalization entails prolonged immobilization and isolation.[13, 14]

Even when excessive use is not attended by significant risk to the patient, it is an indication of poor care on at least two counts: First, it suggests that the physician, if he is responsible for the excessive use, is misinformed or has used poor judgment; second, it constitutes a waste of resources, for not only is overuse wasteful in itself—it also reduces the availability of services to others who might need them.

For these reasons, the present volume will view wasteful or inappropriate use as an element in the appraisal of quality. Utilization review will therefore be considered as one aspect of quality appraisal, with a somewhat different emphasis, but not diverging in any fundamental manner from other forms of quality appraisal.

That the conceptual and operational melding of quality appraisal and utilization review is in keeping with the principles set forth in Medicare regulations is clearly illustrated by the following quotation from *Conditions of Participation for Hospitals*.[15] The quotation also illustrates the emphasis on underuse as well as overuse and points out several dimensions of quality.

> The review plan of a hospital should have as its overall objective the maintenance of high quality patient care, and an increase in effective utilization of hospital services to be achieved through an educational approach involving study of patterns of care, and the encouragement of appropriate utilization. It is contemplated that a review of the medical necessity of admissions and durations of stay, for example, would take into account alternative use and availability of out-of-hospital facilities and services. The review of professional services furnished might include study of such conditions as overuse or underuse of services, logical substantiation of diagnoses, proper use of consultation, and whether required diagnostic workup and treatment are initiated and carried out promptly. Review of lengths of stay might consider not only medical necessity, but the effect that hospital staffing may have on duration of stay, whether assistance is available to the physician in arranging for discharge planning, and the availability of out-of-hospital facilities and services which will assure continuity of care.[15]

Further Development of Material

At this point it may be useful to present to the reader a brief preview of the material in subsequent sections of this volume.

First, there will be a brief description of selected methods of appraisal that will make no clear distinction between those which emphasize content of care and those which emphasize quantity of care. This will be followed by a section devoted to methodological problems in collecting, quantifying and interpreting information. A section will follow covering issues of policy and implementation germane to quality and utilization review in organized medical care settings. The succeeding section will attempt to identify certain areas requiring further research and development. The concluding section of the text will present a brief summary.

A list of references and an annotated bibliography of recent literature are appended.*

A major organizational feature of the book content separates considerations of methodological issues, of policy and of implementation from the description of existing methods of appraisal. These issues are of a basic nature and cut across all or several of the appraisal methods. Organization of the material in this manner therefore diminishes repetition. Perhaps of greater importance, it may contribute to a more thorough grasp of the basic problems and issues in measurement and implementation. This benefit, in turn, may enable the administrator to devise and apply a system of appraisal to his own situation in a more competent and flexible manner than he otherwise might. After all, the objective of this volume of *A Guide to Medical Care Administration* is not solely to equip the administrator to select from among existing methods of appraisal, but to help him construct and develop one best suited to his particular needs.

---

* Further references may be found in a bibliography recently published by the Public Health Service. D. C. Riedel, *Utilization Review: A Selected Bibliography* (Arlington, Virginia, Division of Medical Care Administration, Public Health Service, 1968), 20 pp.

Part II:

SELECTED METHODS OF APPRAISAL

As we have already emphasized, this volume of the Guide is concerned with assuring the quality of care in operating programs. However, it does not deal with all the ways by which assurance of quality may be achieved. It restricts itself to formal review mechanisms which have a specific control function, selecting further from among them only those that have a significant element of appraisal or evaluation. For example, various procedures for verification, authentication and authorization are not considered to qualify as appraisal and are therefore excluded.

Summary of Classification of Methods

The following classification has been adopted for presenting the methods to be described in this section.

1. Appraisal of process
   a. Certification
   b. Statistical display and analysis of patterns of care
   c. Case review
      (1) With implicit criteria
      (2) With explicit criteria
   d. Appraisal of the data used for clinical decision making
2. Appraisal of end results
   a. As a monitoring activity
   b. As a research and evaluation activity

It will soon become evident that this classification is not completely successful in creating mutually exclusive categories. For example, the monitoring of end results can most conveniently be part of a system of statistical display and analysis of patterns of care, which includes type and amount as well as end results. However, the classification is satisfactory in pointing out certain major distinctions.

Appraisal of Process
Certification

Certification, as ordinarily carried out, is perhaps better described as a method of delegated review and control rather than as a method of assessment. Usually the physician in charge is delegated by the program to decide whether care is suitable, and he then certifies its appropriateness. In effect, the physician is being asked to assess the appropriateness of his own care as well as that of the other services he has ordered for his patient. In so doing, he is expected to use his best professional judgment, with or without external guidelines provided by the program. Thus, he exercises not only self-control, but also control over the wishes and propensities of his client, and, in controlling any tendencies for clients to "abuse" the program, he functions, in part, as the agent of the program.

Delegation of the certification function is almost never complete. The decisions of the individual physician are usually subject to review by his colleagues in the provision of care and/or by his peers on behalf of the program that finances care. This review process introduces a larger element of appraisal and it justifies the inclusion of certification as one of the methods to be described in this section.

There are several types of certification, depending on when in the course of care certification is required. Initial certification may take place before, or at the time of, the commencement of care. Subsequent certification may follow, once or repeatedly, at specified intervals. The times for first and subsequent certification may be uniform, being the same for all diseases, conditions or types of care, or they may be variable, being different for each disease, condition or type of care.

Early Medicare regulations offer an excellent example of the requirement for initial certification followed by recertification at uniform intervals:

> Briefly, the requirements are: The attending physician or a member of the medical staff having knowledge of the case must state in writing at the time of admission or as soon thereafter as possible the medical necessity for the hospital admission. The first recertification must be no later than the 14th day of hospitalization. A second recertification is required by the 21st day of hospitalization, with subsequent recertifications as of a lapsed time set by the local utilization review committee but at intervals of no more than 30 days. At the option of the hospital, the utilization review committee's review of extended duration stays can take the place of the third and subsequent recertification.[16]

Certification of hospital stay at a given time which is uniform for all conditions has been a feature of many Blue Cross plans. Tabulation II-1 summarizes the situation in 1965 among 73 plans that responded to a questionnaire:[17]

CERTIFICATION

Tabulation II-1

Days of Stay Before Certification Is Required	Number of Plans
7	1
10	1
14	6
15	4
21	8
30	7
More than 30	3
Total	30

The institution of uniform-interval certification appears to be a fairly well-established procedure in medical care organization. It is therefore surprising to see that no clear rationale for the choice of most appropriate times at which certification is to be sought has been developed. Several studies have shown that long hospital stays are frequently unnecessary. Moreover, although such stays are relatively infrequent, they account for a disproportionate number of unnecessary hospital days. Thus, Rosenfeld *et al.* found, in four Boston hospitals, that 42 percent of patients who, on a given hypothetical day had been in hospital 30 days or longer, did not require active hospital care. Furthermore, although such long stay cases constituted only six percent of discharges, they accounted for 32 percent of hospital days used during the year.[18] A more recent study has shown an essentially similar picture for hospitals in New York City, where nine municipal and voluntary general hospitals were studied. On a given day, 26 percent of patients in municipal hospitals and 21 percent of those in voluntary hospitals were found to have been in hospital for 30 days or longer. Of such patients, 41 percent were judged not to require the services of a general hospital. The proportion of those in hospital unnecessarily was 50 percent for long-stay cases in municipal hospitals. It varied between 15–59 percent for those in voluntary hospitals, with an average of 29 percent.[19]

These figures are cited to indicate the magnitude of the problem and to explain in part why so much attention has been directed, in schemes of utilization review, at the justification for extended hospital stay. Since the problem is even more serious among the elderly, this emphasis in Medicare is easy to understand. But there are those who suggest that the emphasis may be partly misplaced. Fitzpatrick has expressed their opinion as follows:

> Part of the reason for recertification programs is an unspoken feeling that long lengths of stay tend to involve more overuse than short lengths of stay. This may be very far from the case. . . . The recently published *Patterns*

of Patient Care,[20] which is a study of effectiveness of hospital use,[12] indicates that a 14-day cutoff point would miss 95.8 percent of the overstays in appendicitis; 68.9 percent of the overstays in fibromyoma of the uterus; 54.9 percent of the overstays in urinary tract infection; and 37.0 percent of the overstays in diabetes. Actually, there is some reason to believe that long lengths of stay tend to be more clearly appropriate. This is because they are more likely to be complicated cases, which are more likely to be appropriate; and because the patient's resources and coverages tend to run out in the longer time period, and greater economic pressure operates on the less sick patients and their physicians.[21]

The data of Riedel and Fitzpatrick, while insufficient to deflect attention from long-stay cases, serve a useful purpose in highlighting the need for systematic elucidation of the concepts and empirical data that underlie the choice of certification intervals. One needs to determine not only how many cases are found to be inappropriately hospitalized at various intervals after admission, but also how many hospital days would be "saved" if hospitalization were interrupted at the time inappropriate use was detected.* In a subsequent section, the need to consider which time for conducting review is most profitable regarding effort in relation to yield will be discussed.

In view of the problems associated with certification and review at uniform intervals, a great deal of interest has recently centered on methods of variable-interval certification. In these methods, the postadmission certification time differs according to diagnostic category. The assumption is that there is an average appropriate length of stay for each diagnosis, and that cases which stay longer ought to be certified as appropriate and perhaps, in addition, reviewed to determine appropriateness. Less attention has been given to review of cases that stay for periods significantly shorter than the average appropriate length of stay. The model that illustrates an approach to certifying and reviewing length of stay at intervals that vary according to diagnosis is the program of Approval by Individual Diagnosis (AID) instituted by the New Jersey Blue Cross and Blue Shield in collaboration with the Medical Society of New Jersey and the New Jersey Hospital Association.[22, 23]

A program of variable-interval certification, such as AID, may be considered to consist of three parts. These are:

1. institution of standards of length of stay,
2. certification and recertification of hospital stay,
3. review of certification decisions.

---

* The concept of "saved" hospital days is itself one that requires exploration. However, that is a matter beyond the scope of this volume.

DETERMINING STANDARDS

The first part consists in a *determination of the standards* of length of stay which are considered to be permissible for each diagnostic category. The manner in which such standards are determined is critical to an understanding of the nature and significance of this method of control.

The AID standards derive primarily from the opinions held by New Jersey physicians of what is maximum permissible length of stay for specified diagnostic categories. The data were obtained by asking the president of the medical staff of each participating hospital to provide, after consultation with his medical staff, an opinion on the "permissible maximum stay, without complication, [so that] the physician would be able to inform each patient as to the expected maximum duration of hospitalization benefits."† The returns were tabulated and the modal length of stay (the one most frequently cited) was almost always used as the standard for AID use. AID standards are therefore primarily normative in derivation. However, the Blue Cross plan had available to it a detailed statistical analysis of actual lengths of stay by diagnosis for all participating New Jersey hospitals for a recent year (1963). These empirical data were compared with the normative data and in a few cases appropriate adjustments of the standards were made in the light of actual experience.

There are 800 three-digit diagnostic codes in the International Statistical Classification. Length of stay standards were determined, as described above, for the 230 most frequent diagnoses. These accounted for 94 percent of the inpatient claims. The remaining diagnoses were all assigned a maximum permissible length of stay of nine days. The 230 frequent diagnoses were listed according to the International Classification with an indication of the standard maximum permissible length of stay for each. A portion of this listing, in the *Manual of Approved Individual Diagnosis*,[22] is reproduced in Tabulation II-2.

This list illustrates a number of the features of AID standards. One notes the degree of diagnostic specificity in some categories and the lack of specificity in others (for example categories 517 and 527). For certain categories a distinction is made for cases treated medically or surgically, and, frequently, different lengths of stay standards are assigned to the two types or cases. The section of the list reproduced above includes the only instance (hypertrophy of the tonsils and adenoids) where a distinction is made according to age. For all other diagnostic categories, no factors other than type of treatment are recognized to make a difference in the standard. Such additional

---

† Quotations are from the memorandum circulated to the presidents of medical staffs surveyed by Blue Cross.

Tabulation II-2

Code		AID Allowed Days Medical	Surgical
	OTHER DISEASES OF RESPIRATORY SYSTEM (510–527)		
510	Hypertrophy of tonsils and adenoids		
	Under 12 years of age	..	2
	12 years of age and over	..	3
513	Chronic sinusitis	7	6*
514	Deflected nasal septum	..	4
517	Other diseases of upper respiratory tract	..	6
518	Pleurisy	14	..
522	Pulmonary congestion and hypostasis	14	..
527	Other diseases of the lung and pleural cavity	12	12

* When it is not clear whether a case is treated medically or surgically, the standard assigned to the more frequent of the two types of treatment is applicable.

factors may, however, be legitimate reasons for departures from the standards, and may be used to explain requests for extension of hospital stay in the manner described below.

The second part of the AID system is the *certification and recertification* of hospital stay. On admission to the hospital, the patient is assigned (usually by the admissions office) the standard length of stay for the diagnosis that is responsible for admission. When there is more than one diagnosis, and it is not clear which is the one primarily responsible for admission, the shortest applicable length of stay is assigned to the case. There is no need for the patient's physician to become involved in certification unless the patient is still in the hospital one or two days prior to the expiration of the original, and automatic, certification. If the patient is not discharged within this interval, the physician is asked to reconsider the case and, if he feels the patient requires a longer stay, to certify to this effect by filling out an appropriate form giving any change in diagnosis, the approximate number of additional days required, and the reason for the extension. One copy of the form is sent to the Blue Cross plan, another is sent to the utilization review committee of the hospital, and a third remains in the patient's hospital chart. This certification procedure may be repeated once or more at the times indicated by the physician in the prior certification. The length of stay for which the plan pays is only limited by the nature of the insurance benefits under the plan.

The third part of the AID system, and one of critical importance, is the *review of individual physicians' certification decisions*. As already described, copies of recertification forms are sent to the insurance plan and to the hospital utilization review committee. It is expected that the major review and control function will be performed by the utilization review committee and that in this way the hospital staff will collectively control its own practices. "In addition, the Plan will review the completed certification forms and call attention of the hospital utilization committee to cases that seem to merit further investigation. In this way, AID can strengthen utilization committees by pinpointing administrative areas, diagnoses and physicians where review might be valuable." [22]

Certain features of the AID system of certification and review deserve special mention. One is the historical development of the program. Certification was introduced by New Jersey Blue Cross in 1955 with initial approvals for 28 days and additional reapprovals at 21-day intervals. In 1963, the period of initial approval was cut down to 14 days and additional reapprovals were required at 14-day intervals.[24] Approval by Individual Diagnosis was introduced in 1965. That this progression may foreshadow a pattern of more general applicability is suggested by Blue Cross data, which show a trend toward shorter approval and reapproval intervals.[17, 21]

Another interesting aspect of the AID program is the convergence of forces that brought about its institution. These included public concern over increasing hospital cost and direct pressure from the insurance commissioner that something be done; shortage of hospital beds in the face of a trend toward longer hospital stays; fruitful collaborative relationships among the Blue plans, the medical society and the hospital association; and strong endorsement by organized labor.[22, 23, 25]

A third feature of some significance is the manner selected to bring pressure to bear upon the physician to comply with the certification procedure. Theoretically, the physician is free not to participate. However, should he refuse to recertify additional days of stay at the expiration of the initial standard period, the patient is informed of this and billed directly for the additional days. Hence, the certification procedure is an attempt to introduce a reciprocal set of controls into the patient-physician relationship. The physician can use the certification requirements to restrain the patient's desire for hospitalization beyond the point of medical necessity, while the patient, pursuing his economic interests, can exert pressure on the physician to cooperate with an essentially administrative process of control. Donabedian and Attwood have pointed out that the control of patients through their physicians, and of physicians through their patients, exemplify frequent approaches in administrative control where the financing agency has no means of exercising more direct controls over the parties concerned. Whether such controls are effective remains to be demonstrated.[26] The effectiveness of this particular method of control as incorporated in AID will be described in a subsequent section of this volume.

A fourth feature is the provision for review while the patient is still in the hospital, enabling the utilization committee, through proper channels, to assist the physician and administrator in achieving more appropriate length of stay.[23a] The significance of such concurrent review, as contrasted with the more usual retrospective review, will be discussed later on in this volume.

Additional features of significance will be commented upon and amplified in subsequent sections. The site of responsibility for utilization control and the appropriate degree of delegation of this responsibility to the managing physician and/or a group of physicians outside the financing agency will be covered at that time. The manner in which standards of length of stay are determined will be part of a more detailed discussion of standard-setting in general.

Statistical Display and Analysis

The introduction of mechanical data-handling systems and, more recently, of computers has made it possible to process, display and summarize large masses of data which are relevant to the administrative appraisal and control of utilization and quality. This specific application was probably pioneered (with initial support by the Kellogg Foundation) by the Commission on Professional and Hospital Activities (CPHA) in Ann Arbor, Michigan. CPHA is a non-profit agency, established in 1955, and sponsored by the American College of Physicians, the American College of Surgeons, the American Hospital Association and the Southwestern Michigan Hospital Council. Its subscriber hospitals, of which there are over 1200, are offered a variety of services, including the Professional Activity Study (PAS), the Medical Audit Program (MAP) and the Length of Stay Package.[27-29] A more recent example, partly patterned on PAS, is the Hospital Utilization Review Project (HUP), cosponsored by the Allegheny County Medical Society Foundation and the Hospital Council of Western Pennsylvania, and supported by the Blue Cross of Western Pennsylvania.[30-32] Methods used by these two agencies (CPHA and HUP) will be the model for the description of statistical display and analysis. However, the intent is to convey a sense of the general applicability of this approach rather than to endorse specific models.

The critical components of a system of statistical display and analysis are:

1. information suitable for mechanical or electronic processing,

STATISTICAL DISPLAY

2. data display and summarization,
3. evaluation.

The basis for a fully-fledged system of statistical display and analysis is, generally, an abstract of each patient's hospital record prepared in such a way as to permit easy coding and transcription for machine or computer processing. The nature and amount of information abstracted from the record, and available for processing, may vary widely. The PAS abstract, for example, has extensive information on patient management, including details of diagnostic work-up and therapy. There are about 150 possible items of information in all. By contrast, HUP uses a much simpler abstract with attention focused mainly on length of stay parameters by type of operation and diagnosis. These parameters include, in addition to total length of stay, the number of days before and after operation or delivery. Thus, the components of the total length of stay are subject to examination.

The statistical system is not necessarily restricted to information in the patient's record. It is possible to set up a system that mechanically combines information from a number of sources so that more elaborate analyses can be made. Such additional data, stored in the computer until called upon, can include more detailed information concerning subscribers as well as physician and hospital characteristics.

The information in both PAS and HUP abstracts tends to concentrate on documenting length of stay and elements of management (professional activities) for type of patient—categorized by diagnosis and by nature of surgical intervention, if any. There are, however, a number of items of intermediate and ultimate end results. These include death or survival, the occurrence of hospital infection or other complications, the removal of diseased or normal tissue at operation, transfer to other hospital or extended care facility, and discharge with approval or against advice. These systems, therefore, do lend themselves to monitoring "outcomes" such as these.

An important feature of both PAS and HUP is that a number of hospitals use a central service for the processing and display of data. The abstracts of individual records are prepared in the hospital, usually by the medical record librarian, and sent to the central agency: Commission on Professional and Hospital Activities and Western Pennsylvania Blue Cross, respectively. Since each PAS and HUP abstract is said to require only five minutes to fill, the amount of work required of the hospital itself is not excessive.[28, 31]

The centralization of data processing, display and analysis results in efficient operations. The central agency can develop expertise, assume leadership in developing new techniques, and engage in promotional and educational activities. Upon request, the agency can help the individual hospital evaluate the findings pertaining to it. The agency can also, within limits set by its own policies, evaluate general patterns of care and disseminate information concerning methods and findings. Finally, the accumulation of a large amount of information in one location makes it possible to summarize patterns of care for a large number of cases so that empirical standards might be constructed and comparisons made among individual or categories of institutions or physicians. For example, the Commission of Professional and Hospital Activities had in 1968 more than 1200 subscribing hospitals and a library of over 36 million case abstracts. Unfortunately for persons with research interests, these hospitals are not a representative cross section because participation is voluntary. The information is valuable nevertheless, and can be put to many administrative and research uses. According to Slee, an increasing number of investigators using the PAS data bank are quite satisfied with projections they are able to make by the use of weighting techniques.[27a]

Data display and summarization is the second major component in the system of statistical appraisal. The advantages of centralizing this activity for a large number of hospitals have already been pointed out. These advantages should be carefully considered before a hospital decides to conduct this activity using its own data-processing equipment and staff.

The first mode of display is to supply listings of cases and of their attributes so that each row provides a coded description of the characteristics and management of each case. To facilitate review, the cases may be arranged in a variety of ways. They may be listed by diagnostic category, by type of operation, by hospital service, by physician, or by combinations of these. Within each category, cases may be ordered by length of stay to permit easier identification of aberrant cases. Aberrant cases may be identified and listed separately. Thus, there may be a separate listing for deaths, for cases with operative complications, or for cases in which certain examinations were not performed. Cases falling below or above certain percentiles of a frequency distribution (of length of stay, for example) can be similarly identified and listed.

In addition to listings, there can be tabulations that summarize experience for a hospital, a hospital department, a physician or surgeon, a diagnostic category, an operative procedure, an age group, and so on. The dependent variable (case characteristic) can be presented in several forms: numbers, frequency distributions, means, percentages, percentiles, and so forth. As might be expected, a large variety of cross tabulations are possible. In some cases, certain indexes may be constructed. For example, PAS has constructed a "variety index" that indicates the number of tests done in the management

EVALUATION

of a case or group of cases, and an "impact index" which weights the number of tests done by a score representing the amount of labor required for each test.[33]

The variety of listings and tabulations described above is intended to give an impression of extreme flexibility and adaptability to particular needs. Needless to say, not all these listings and tabulations are routinely available. Both PAS and HUP provide a limited number of routine listings and tables. However, special analyses may be undertaken for special purposes.

Evaluation is the third major component of a statistical system of appraisal. It is usual to say that a statistical system merely presents data in a form suitable for rapid perusal and evaluation by the expert administrator and physician. For example, the Commission on Professional and Hospital Activities is very careful to point out that its role is merely "to increase the accessibility of information contained in medical records so that it can be used to greater advantage in the improvement of patient care."[28] This is true, but only in part. In selecting items of information for inclusion in the system, in presenting and analyzing data, and in providing bench marks and comparative data, the statistical system helps direct evaluation into certain channels, thereby influencing it. But the final decision as to whether what shows up in the statistical material is "good" or "bad," acceptable or unacceptable, remains with the hospital and its staff.

The appropriate hospital authorities interpret the patterns of care in their hospital by using commonly accepted notions of what is suitable care. Questions may be raised about the diagnosis of myocardial infarction without the performance of certain diagnostic tests, about reports of positive laboratory tests without evidence of follow-up, or concerning excessively long stays without apparent reason deducible from the data in the abstract. All these judgments involve the application of accepted notions of what is good practice (normative standards).

Statistical data also lend themselves to comparisons among physicians and institutions, and the identification of deviance from the average for a group of physicians or institutions. This is the unique contribution of evaluation by statistical display and analysis. Further refinements can be made by comparing like with like. PAS uses various characteristics to group hospitals in a manner most suited to the question at hand. Hospitals are frequently grouped by number of discharges into four categories: small, medium small, medium large, and large. Other classificatory criteria include teaching status, facilities available and geographic location.[27a] Shindell believes that an important feature of HUP is the comparison of all hospitals in a community.[30] Slee emphasizes the usefulness of PAS in making possible comparisons between practice in the hospitals of a given community with practice in other communities.[27a]

The potential of such comparisons can be seen in some of the following examples. The HUP program prepares hospital "profiles" which show graphically the rank of each hospital, within an array of all hospitals in the community, in average length of stay for a number of selected medical and surgical conditions, further indicating whether the hospital has risen or fallen in rank since the previous time period. The CPHA "Length of Stay Package" shows the average length of stay by diagnostic category in a given hospital, the average length of stay for matching patients in a standard population of discharges, the difference between each pair of lengths of stay, and whether the difference is significant.[28] This CPHA tabulation is based on a method that permits standardization of length of stay by diagnosis, age, whether an operation has been performed and whether there is a secondary diagnosis.[29, 34] Such comparative studies constitute the application of empirical standards, and represent the major contribution of a method of statistical display and analysis to evaluation.

Certain aspects of evaluation through statistical display and analysis deserve special mention. To begin with a technical point, it is important to examine frequency distributions, as well as averages, when evaluating the data. (In a subsequent section there will be mention of problems of sample size and sampling variation.)

A second point is to emphasize that deviation from the statistical average does not automatically mean something is wrong. The average should not be equated with the good. Deviations merely draw attention to phenomena that may require more careful examination.

A third issue is the nature of primary emphasis in the system: whether on quality or on utilization. We have already indicated that the primary emphasis in HUP is on justification of admission and length of stay. By contrast, PAS–MAP includes consideration of many more aspects of management. In light of the previous discussion of definitions of quality in this volume, the difference may be seen as one of degree rather than kind. Concern with length of stay may be considered to represent interest in one of the many dimensions of quality. As more information is collected and evaluated, the appraisal of quality becomes multidimensional and therefore more meaningful and definitive.

A fourth issue is whether the purpose of evaluation is to identify individual error or wrongdoing, or to discover institutional patterns that require changes in administrative procedure or organization. Which approach is emphasized depends in part on what one believes explains medical behavior in organizations. Shindell has stressed

25

EVALUATION

that length of stay in a hospital is determined partly by accepted modes of practice shared by the majority of the medical staff, and partly by administrative and organizational features of pervasive influence over which the individual physician has limited control. Excessive average lengths of stay are rarely said to be the doing of a few "offenders." Hence the emphasis in analysis and action is on institutional performance rather than the performance of the individual physician.[25, 30, 31] On the other hand, analysis of PAS data has clearly disclosed aberrant physician, as well as institutional, behavior, indicating the need to observe the practice of individual physicians in addition to that of institutions.[35] Needless to say, the two approaches, far from being mutually exclusive, are reciprocally reinforcing. It is apparent that individual performance should be observed and studied. The group behavior of physicians, and the administrative and organizational factors that influence this behavior, are also of importance. Choice of emphasis in any given situation is often a matter of policy and strategy.

Finally, it should be clear that statistical display and analysis is often only a step in an evaluative sequence, and does not represent the entire sequence. Often, the next step consists of a more intensive study of case records, as the statistical system may reveal pervasive patterns that require investigation and correction. An unusually long average preoperative stay may bring about the examination of a representative sample of cases in order to determine the reason, which may be insufficient preadmission work-up, delays in ordering tests or receiving their results, or problems of scheduling in the operating room. Shindell has emphasized that the study of cases will often lead to further administrative and organizational studies designed to elucidate the problem and bring about appropriate action. The HUP program is, in fact, seen to include the more extensive sequence indicated in the following steps: [31]

> Abstracting the medical record in a form suitable for automatic data processing,
> Using data processing to compile statistics on hospital use,
> Summarizing comparative experience for specific categories of patients,
> Constructing a profile for a hospital by reflecting comparative experience in a number of diagnostic categories,
> Instituting case reviews in the specific areas of abnormal experience to identify practices and procedures deserving further investigation,
> Performing special studies of administrative and professional practices and procedures where indicated (p. 7).

A similar sequence of activities can be said to characterize the PAS system, with the exception of step 6. PAS does not offer to go into hospitals to perform special administrative studies such as HUP made of operating room scheduling.[27a]

In addition to revealing undesired patterns of care, the statistical system will also precisely identify the aberrant cases so that attention can be focused on these. One use, therefore, of the statistical system is as a screen to identify those cases that require more detailed review by the audit committee, utilization review committee or other appropriate authority within the hospital.

Case Review

The review of clinical charts constitutes the most detailed examination of professional performance in systems for the appraisal of quality and use of service. In one sense case review is the most definitive of all methods of assessment; and yet it suffers from a variety of defects which shall be discussed in subsequent sections of this volume.

Case review may be carried out externally by one or more examiners who are independent of the hospital, or internally by one or more committees of the medical staff itself. One may thus distinguish two kinds of audit: external and internal.

A further classification hinges on the degree to which the standards and procedures for evaluation have been formalized and made explicit. According to one approach, the reviewing physician, or group, examines the record and then judges whether the case has been appropriately managed. The examiners function essentially as expert physicians who vicariously manage the case as it is revealed in the record and compare actual management against what would have been, hypothetically, their own. Models of this approach are the studies of quality conducted by the Columbia University School of Public Health and Administrative Medicine for the Teamsters' Union [38-40] and, to a lesser extent, those of the Health Insurance Plan of Greater New York.[36, 37]

The second approach is characterized by prior explicit and formal specification of the criteria and procedures to be used in evaluation. The reviewers must still use their professional judgment, but their discretion is somewhat limited by instructions as to what aspects of care they should consider and by some specification of the appropriate basis for arriving at certain diagnoses or performing certain procedures. They are also sometimes instructed as to the kinds of procedures indicated or contraindicated in particular situations. The work of Lembcke constitutes an early model of this second approach.[41-43] Lembcke developed the criteria as guides for his own use in external audits which he performed at the invitation of hospitals. A more recent model, which Payne developed and designated

APPRAISAL OF DATA

as the "criteria approach" to evaluation, may be seen as an extension of Lembcke's work. Payne's model differs, however, in at least two significant respects: It is an internal audit rather than an external one. The criteria are developed by, or through, active participation of the medical staff of the hospital. This means that the medical staff have reached agreement on the standards, know what they are, and expect to be judged by them.[44-47]

While it may be useful to distinguish two types of case review by the extent to which criteria and procedures are formally specified, it may be misleading to call one of the two types the "criteria approach." The distinction is not one of criteria versus no criteria, but of implicit versus explicit criteria. While the second type could be called the "explicit criteria" approach, the reader must realize that the distinctions are not sharp. There is a continuum between a minimum of specification at one end and complete specification at the other. The degree of specification in the "criteria approach" is, in fact, quite modest and far from complete.

It is also evident that the explicit specification of criteria is a characteristic that may apply equally to external and internal audits. In fact, the "criteria approach" developed by Payne is based on a survey technique first devised to study the appropriateness of length of stay in Michigan hospitals.[12]

In subsequent sections of this volume there will be a more detailed discussion of the many methodological and policy issues that pertain to the assessment of quality in general. Since these are particularly relevant to case review, it would be repetitious to dwell upon them at this point.

Appraisal of the Data Used for Clinical Decision Making

The quality of patient management depends upon the completeness and veracity of the data which form the basis for the physician's diagnostic and therapeutic decisions. Determining whether the physician obtains the necessary information to manage any given case properly is an integral part of the appraisal of process by statistical display and analysis of patterns of care and, especially, by case review. But little attention has been given to checks on the veracity of the data, such as physical findings or laboratory and diagnostic tests, that are used in making decisions. Generally, the data are assumed to be valid and assessment is based on whether the appropriate data have been obtained and the proper inferences drawn from them. However, the judges would expect the managing physician to question the veracity of the data with which he works whenever inconsistencies are apparent to the assessor, or in situations where the prudent physician would be expected to seek confirmation. This orientation is appropriate if the concern of the assessment is with the ability of the physician to obtain and logically manipulate medical evidence. Conversely, it can be asserted that patient management cannot be of high quality if the physician has to work with inaccurate primary data.

A considerable literature attests to the frequency of observer error in the evaluation of physical signs and the interpretation of diagnostic evidence such as X-ray films, electrocardiographic tracings and pathological specimens.[48] In one hospital, Lembcke found the true incidence of uterine hyperplasia to be between five and eight percent rather than 60 to 65 percent of uterine curettages, as reported by the hospital pathologist.[41] Schaeffer's study of laboratories in New York City has revealed considerable deficiencies in their ability to identify accurately specimens of known characteristics submitted to them.[49] About a third of laboratories were rated unsatisfactory in both bacteriology and chemistry. Only seven percent of laboratories were rated "consistently good" in both bacteriology and chemistry.

This study of New York City laboratories attempted to examine the relationship between structure and the accuracy of laboratory tests. It was found that about 22 percent of municipal hospitals were rated "consistently good" in both bacteriology and chemistry, whereas only about one percent of independent hospitals were so rated. "Attempts were made to relate the quality of performance to the education and experience of directors, the education and number of supervisory personnel, the number of annual tests and the types of laboratories. It was concluded that all those laboratories which consistently perform well were staffed with highly trained, on site, supervisors."[49]

Such findings demonstrate that neither the physician interested in the welfare of his patient, nor the administrator concerned with the effectiveness of his program, can afford to ignore the possibility of inaccuracies in the primary data on which diagnosis and therapy are based. The discoveries reported by Schaeffer indicate that steps exist which can be taken to organize the laboratory service so as to increase accuracy in test results. These steps, though essential, are not the subject of our concern in this volume. What we must confront is the question of how to keep under surveillance the accuracy of the primary data used in diagnosis and treatment.

The validity of the physician's interpretation of physical signs is a matter of great importance in his clinical performance. His interpretive capacity may be evaluated under special test situations.[50, 51] However, it must be recognized that this aspect of performance has

29

APPRAISAL OF DATA

seldom, if ever, been part of an established system of quality assessment.

The validity of laboratory tests may be checked by independent examination of the material submitted for testing or interpretation. The examination may be part of a general assessment of the quality of the medical care process. For example, the hospital audits conducted by Lembcke included reexamination of diagnostic evidence (films, tracings, slides) by competent judges.[41] The verification of laboratory test results may also be a separate, self-contained activity conducted internally by the program itself, or externally by some competent supervisory agency. An illustration of external verification is Schaeffer's description of the methods used by the New York City Department of Health to watch over the performance of clinical laboratories in the City.[49] About four times a year each laboratory receives specimens, of known characteristics, to examine by means of microbiology, chemistry, syphilis serology, cross matching and hemoglobin determination. The performance of each laboratory is compared with that of at least two reference laboratories in each specialty. The specimens to be tested are delivered by Health Department examiners who personally observe the testing procedures in each laboratory.

In addition to, or in place of, a direct check on the reproducibility and validity of diagnostic tests, persistent and significant inaccuracies in primary data may cause adverse end results that come to light through end result monitoring or review. Aberrant patterns of laboratory findings, or of care, may also alert the administrator that something is wrong. A classic example has been culled from the reports of the Professional Activity Study. A study of average admission hemoglobin values in 66 hospitals, in four categories of hospital size, showed a degree of variability that could not be fully explained by interhospital differences in altitude, age or sex of patient or types of clinical material treated in the several hospitals. It was concluded that the amount of variation could not be explained unless laboratory bias was considered.[52] A subsequent study at one hospital did, in fact, show improper standardization of the hemoglobin measuring instrument that resulted in uniformly lower readings. Elimination of this bias increased the average reported hemoglobin value in this hospital by 1.5 grams per 100 milliliters. This increase was paralleled by a drop in blood usage of over one thousand pints a year and an estimated yearly reduction in hospital costs of $25,000.[53]

A centralized statistical display and analysis system that includes data on laboratory findings permits a study of variability and secular trends within a given hospital as well as among participating hospitals. This can provide early warning of possible systematic error in laboratory reports and serve as a safeguard additional to whatever methods of standardization and replication are in force in the laboratory.

Appraisal of End Results

We have referred to the appraisal of end results (or outcomes) as one of the three basic approaches to assessment, mentioned the tendency of preference to be polarized in favor of either process or end result, speculated on what accounts for this polarization, and indicated the need to include both process and end results in systems of continuous or repeated appraisal. This section will further discuss the definitions and classification of end results, the uses and limitations of end results as indicators of the quality of medical care, and some operational aspects of end result appraisal.

The first problem is deciding what an end result (or outcome) is. According to Shapiro, "The term 'end result' refers to some measurable aspect of health status which is influenced by a particular element, or array of . . . elements of medical care."[54] Shapiro's definition thus focuses on changes in the person or unit, a family for example, that is the identifiable object of care. Presumably the change should be of sufficient magnitude and duration to be significant and, to permit use in appraisal, it should be measurable. Deciding what kinds of changes are relevant is limited only by one's definition of "health" and by the objectives of that portion of the health care system which is under evaluation. End results take into account the physical structure and physiological function of the person or unit, as well as psychological and social performance. Examples of end result evaluation assembled by Shapiro are: general mortality and longevity, perinatal mortality, case fatality, survival curves in chronic conditions including cancer, acute and chronic morbidity, presence of symptoms and signs, severity and frequency of illness, physical disability, complications of pregnancy, birth weight, the Apgar score of newborn health,[55] loss of time from school or work, work modification, unemployment or ability to continue at work, modification in activities of daily living, changes in family composition, degree of self-care, sleep and rest patterns, personal hygiene, habits and recreational activity.

Sanazaro and Williamson have recently attempted to supply a classification of end results deduced from descriptions of "critical incidents" cited by internists to illustrate "effective" and "ineffective" episodes of care.[56, 57] This classification is not meant to provide a complete coverage of all categories of end results at which one might arrive inductively, but is of particular interest because it indicates what aspects of end results are salient in the minds of a selected

31

group of unusually competent internists engaged in both clinical practice and teaching. It also illustrates the multiple dimensions that may be subsumed under the definition of "quality" as viewed by the physician. (See section on Frame of Reference.)

- A. Patient end results
  1. Life saved, death caused
     a. Length of life
  2. Physical abnormalities
     a. Diseases, states, conditions and their complications
     b. Anatomical abnormalities (signs)
     c. Physiological abnormalities (signs)
     d. Biochemical abnormalities (signs)
  3. Psychological abnormalities
     Psychiatric syndromes, e.g., schizophrenia, or psychological entities, e.g., cardiac neurosis
  4. Physical symptoms
     Subjective complaints of patient caused by biological abnormalities, e.g., pain, dizziness, weakness, anxiety, depression
  5. Psychological symptoms
     Subjective complaints of patients caused by emotional problems
  6. Function
     Functioning of patient as an individual (self-care, work, school), as a member of a family (role as parent or mate), as a member of society (community, church).
- B. Process outcomes
  7. Attitudes toward physician and care received
     Attitudes and feelings such as trust, confidence, satisfaction toward M.D. or episode of care
  8. Attitudes toward understanding of condition responsible for episode of care
  9. Compliance
     Patient's diligence in following physician's instructions about medication, diet, activity, habits, follow-up and continuity of care with same M.D.
  10. Risks and unnecessary procedures
      Potentially harmful or unnecessary procedures, tests, surgery
  11. Hospitalization
      Duration, frequency, appropriateness
  12. Cost
      Direct expenditures or loss of income

Certain features of this classification are noteworthy. The distinction between "patient end results" and "process outcomes" is based on the fact that the outcomes in the second category occur only when the patient receives medical care, whereas the end results in the first category are not uniquely dependent on medical intervention. The process outcomes also seem to extend the notion of end results to cover phenomena—risks and unnecessary procedures, hospitalization and costs—that are not clearly changes in the recipient himself or in his behavior. The significance of this enlargement of the definition of end results will be further discussed below.

Another interesting aspect of the classification is the range of end results considered by physicians to be both significant and relevant to medical care and physician performance. It is important to note, however, that "process outcomes" appear to be less salient than "patient end results." "Patient end results" accounted for 70 percent of all outcomes cited. In fact, 61 percent of all items cited were accounted for by four categories of "patient end results": longevity, physical abnormalities, psychological symptoms and "functions." Conspicuously absent is the category of access to care. This illustrates clearly the distinctions in level and scope of concern that were made in the earlier section of this volume entitled "Frame of Reference."

Shapiro further enlarges the scope of end result appraisal by indicating that end results may be assessed indirectly, as well as directly. The indirect approach consists in measuring, or identifying the presence or absence of, those elements of care that have a known relationship, whether favorable or unfavorable, to end results. This extension appears reasonable from the viewpoint of an organization providing care to a definable population group. Such an organization must be concerned with the extent to which it provides access to persons most in need of care, achieves the use of screening or other preventive services by its clients, engages in follow-up of questionable findings, accomplishes early institution of prenatal care, and so on. These activities are, in one sense, organizational products and are presumed to make a contribution to the recipient's health and well-being. Furthermore, it is reasonable for those who define their organizational objectives in terms of outcomes, expressed as client health and well-being, to consider elements of process as indirect evidence of good or bad outcome. It is equally reasonable, as Donabedian has pointed out, for those who define organizational objectives in terms of process to consider outcomes as indirect evidence that good or bad care has been provided.[58]

However, the proposals that end results can be indirectly measured by process, and process indirectly measured by end results, do lead to a confusing situation. Clarification comes from the study of organizations, a field where the definition of means and ends has posed a similar problem. The solution proposed by Simon is to consider the entire spectrum of activities or events as a chain in which each link is an outcome of a previous link and a means to the one that follows.[59] Several authors have pointed out that this formulation provides a useful approach to evaluation.[60-62] It could also help resolve the problem of whether one is evaluating process or outcomes. To do so, a description of the chain of events that is under consideration and a

33

specification of the link or links in the chain that are being appraised would be necessary. The model of the medical care process proposed by Donabedian could be used in this way.[5]

The words "process" and "outcome" or "end result" are convenient, and will continue to be used. It is proposed, therefore, that "outcome" or "end result" be restricted to designate states of structure or function in the recipient. These are almost always states of health and well-being, even though it is recognized that health itself may be a means to a further objective.

Certain antecedents of outcome constitute focal end points for evaluation, and may be designated as "procedural end points"[1] or intermediate outcomes. For example, the percent of persons diagnosed as having pneumonia who receive a chest X-ray may be considered a measure of a procedural end point. The percent of primary appendectomies in which pathological examination shows normal tissue might be called an intermediate outcome.

What are the uses and advantages of end results as indicators of the quality of medical care? The most important and distinctive advantage is their considerable, and seldom questioned, degree of face validity as a dimension of quality. Good and bad outcomes are generally culturally defined. Therefore, the values that govern them are pervasive, agreed upon and relatively stable. In fact, most aspects of process are subject to validation by observation of how they contribute to outcomes. This should be completely true for the purely technical components of management. All professional norms concerning technical management are derived from demonstrated or presumed relationships between management actions and end results expressed as health and well-being. Thus, the first use of end results is their validating function.

The second use may be called their integrative function. Since end results represent the net effect of the operation of many factors and processes, they reflect the contributions not only of care rendered by physicians, but by other health professionals as well. Similarly, during any one episode of illness, all components of care, whether ambulatory or inpatient, contribute to ultimate outcome. The many disparate strands and components of care, which are difficult or impossible to evaluate separately, converge, as it were, in some definable outcome which represents them collectively. There is further summation over time, so that the health of an individual at a given moment reflects the effect of care throughout a lifetime. The generations may even be bridged, as when a newborn's health is influenced by the health care received by the mother during her own childhood.

The third use of end results may be called their innovative function. A study of end results often raises the question, why? Why, for example, are mortality and morbidity rates in one hospital or program different from those in another? Observed differences in outcome lead to studies of antecedents and bring about knowledge of what are desirable elements in the organization and delivery of care.[54]

Finally, end results tend to be concrete, and therefore seemingly amenable to fairly precise measurement. This is certainly true for variables such as mortality and longevity, and reasonably true for states of morbidity and disability. Behavioral and attitudinal variables may be more difficult to define and measure. While there is considerable experience in the measurement of outcome, a review of this experience, though germane to the present volume, is beyond its rather modest scope. Brief reference to some methods of outcome measurement may, however, be of value to the reader.

At the community level, Dorn provides a useful summary of morbidity concepts basic to measurement.[63] The publications of the National Center for Health Statistics, especially those in *Series 2*, provide much useful information concerning the concepts and methods of measuring morbidity and use of health services in the population by interview surveys and screening examinations.[64,65] An early publication of the World Health Organization deals with various approaches to the measurement of population health.[66] Feldman provides an excellent evaluative review of household interview surveys.[67] Two papers by Sanders give a thought-provoking critique of present approaches and suggest some new ones.[68,69]

At the individual level, some ingenious methods have been developed for measuring the effects of rehabilitation services.[70-72] Rice *et al.* describe some simple indices for measuring the outcome of mental hospital care.[73] There is a considerable literature in the measurement of mental health and evaluation of the effects of psychotherapy.[74-76]

In order to use end result appraisal effectively it is necessary to understand clearly several important limitations. The most significant of these arises from one of the major virtues of end results: their capacity to integrate. Since end results represent the combined effect of many factors, including those unrelated to medical care, it is often difficult to determine the extent to which a certain outcome is attributable to medical care. For example, it is difficult to say to what extent differences in levels of perinatal mortality among countries, population groups, or institutions are attributable to differences in the quality of medical care. Many factors in addition to medical care influence health and well-being: age, sex, race, geographic location, occupation, education, income, nutrition and housing. What makes the situation even more complex is that these factors exert their effect directly, as well as indirectly, through the availability and

END RESULTS

use of health services. The impact of all factors, other than medical care, which influence outcome must be accounted for before the residual effect attributed to medical care itself can be determined. Assuming this can be done, it may still be difficult to say precisely what aspect of medical care is responsible for the favorable or unfavorable outcomes observed.

These difficulties account for the frequent use of comparisons of specified populations in end result appraisal. Observed differences in end result can then be attributed to the characteristics that are dissimilar. But it is difficult to design studies in which similarities and differences are clearly, reliably and completely identified.

Assessment requires standards. Unfortunately, end result standards are usually not easy to specify. There is considerable agreement on what constitutes a good end result; but there is little knowledge on how good an end result can be achieved in a particular situation even if the best medical care is applied. Normative end result standards are, therefore, poorly developed, which is another reason for using comparisons in end result studies. Comparisons will not be as necessary when there is sufficient knowledge about the natural history of disease, and about the capabilities of medicine to permit specification of the anticipated effect of medical intervention in designated disease situations.[54] The utility of end result appraisal will increase as knowledge accumulates concerning the relationship between process and outcome, and between structure and outcome.

Another limitation in end result appraisal is the time taken for certain end results to occur. Many years may elapse before the effect of management on certain diseases becomes firmly established. While the researcher may be able to wait for such results to become manifest, the administrator needs early feedback in order to assess the effectiveness of his operations. M. Sheps has pointed out that long lags may also seriously handicap the researcher, because the comparability of groups under observation is progressively lost as new and different factors enter the situation (Reference 6, page 89).

Ease of measurement may appear as one advantage of end result appraisal. It is not always true that end results are concrete and easy to measure. There may be considerable difficulties in the definition of outcomes and their measurement. Sullivan has discussed some of the problems of measuring health.[77] Kelman and Willner point out some of the difficulties encountered in evaluating the effects of rehabilitation services.[78]

We have emphasized that accepted validity is the major strength of end result assessment. However, even this is open to certain limitations, partly because medical care may alter the natural history of disease so as to produce unexpected and seemingly paradoxical effects. Sanders has noted that better medical care may result in higher age-specific morbidity rates.[69] He attributes this in part to the survival of disease-prone persons who might have died earlier in the absence of good medical care. This problem of morbidity-mortality interaction may be handled by constructing an index of health that combines morbidity and mortality.[79] The index may then be used to determine the days of life lost or saved for specified population cohorts.

At least part of the increase in morbidity reported in a population receiving higher levels of care may be spurious. It may result from greater propensity to seek care and greater opportunities for the diagnosis of illness.[69, 80]

Another qualification on the validity of outcomes is the need to interpret them within the context of the appropriate culture or subculture. For example, McDermott *et al.* have observed that fixing a congenitally dislocated hip joint in a given position is considered good medicine for the white man; but it can prove crippling for the Navajo Indian who spends much time seated on the floor or in the saddle.[81]

Finally, relevant outcomes should be selected for evaluation. For example, recovery may not be a reasonable expectation in certain illnesses. Instead, the prolongation of useful life, or the reduction of pain and discomfort, may be the relevant outcome. In other situations recovery is the rule; reassurance and the reduction of anxiety may be the appropriate outcome to measure.

A recent study of perinatal mortality in two Air Force hospitals illustrates vividly both the uses and limitations of end result evaluation. The investigators began by assuming that the populations receiving care at the two hospitals were reasonably comparable and that differences in perinatal mortality would be more likely to reflect differences in the quality of care. When they tested their assumption, they found out that even in this situation there were significant differences in race, age of mother, parity and receipt of prenatal care—all factors known to be related to perinatal mortality. When these factors were taken into account, there were still differences in perinatal mortality in the two hospitals. These findings raise most dramatically the question of what accounts for these differences, but provide no direct information on the quality of medical care. The authors speculate as follows concerning some of the determinants of outcome in this study:

> Why was Hospital A unable to accomplish the same results in the care of Negro dependents as it accomplished in white patients? Why was the white primipara perinatal mortality and submaturity experience in Hospital B substantially above that found in Hospital A? Why were the perinatal mortality

MONITORING

and submaturity rates so high among Oriental mothers married to Caucasian husbands? Unfortunately, these questions cannot be answered at this time. Quality control measurements only tell us whether certain values are aberrant, thus indicating whether further study is warranted.[82]

A discussion of the limitations of end result appraisal does not imply that end results are not useful indicators of the quality of medical care. On the contrary, the intent of the discussion is to show precisely what end results have to contribute to evaluation, and to permit the administrator to use them properly and effectively.

On the question of implementation, there are at least three ways in which end result assessment becomes a part of an operational system of quality appraisal and control: (1) creation of a system to monitor outcomes; (2) case analysis of outcomes, usually unfavorable ones; and (3) special studies with a research orientation.

End result monitoring depends on selecting certain critical end results which are considered to reflect the performance of professionals in patient care or the effectiveness of the medical care system as a whole. Precisely what outcomes are chosen depends on the frame of reference within which evaluation proceeds, the hypothetical relationships between a given end result and the process elements that contribute to it, and the availability of information and the amenability of the end result to reliable measurement.

The rationale of the end result monitoring system is that under acceptable conditions of operation a certain level of adverse end results is expected. Any significant deviation from this expected level calls for immediate investigation to determine what is responsible. (Considerations that go into determining what is an "expected" or "acceptable" level and what constitutes "significant deviation" will be discussed in a subsequent section.)

The end result monitoring system may stand on its own. One example is the "alerter system" described by Bundesen.[83] Introduced and operated by the health department in Chicago, this system obtains, tabulates and displays current reports on infant deaths below seven days of age in all Chicago hospitals. It is possible, by referring to appropriate display panels, to compare current data for each hospital with previous data for that same hospital. It is also possible to compare data from one hospital with data from each of the other hospitals in Chicago, and to find the average for all of them. Increase in the rate of first-week deaths, or the occurrence of seemingly preventable deaths, is a signal for investigation and corrective action. More often, end result monitoring is part and parcel of a statistical analysis and display system that keeps under surveillance a variety of "procedural end points," "intermediate outcomes" and "end results."

The second operational approach to end result assessment is *case review and analysis of unfavorable outcomes.* Again, this may stand independently or be linked to a system of statistical display and analysis. End result monitoring obviously requires case analysis when tolerance limits are exceeded. However, the decision may be made that the tolerance for certain outcomes is zero and that every instance of such outcomes, or a representative sample of them, should be examined to determine how they may be prevented. In certain instances it may be also necessary to assign responsibility for failure. For example, all maternity, perinatal and postoperative deaths may be subject to this kind of detailed scrutiny.

The analysis of unfavorable outcomes has been a remarkably effective research and operational tool. A notable example is the study of perinatal deaths conducted under the auspices of the New York Academy of Medicine.[84] This was an analysis by a committee of expert physicians of the medical records pertaining to a sample of perinatal deaths. The committee identified preventable aspects in each death and assigned responsibility for such aspects to the physician or the client. In addition, it investigated relationships of certain factors to outcome and preventability, including the type of hospital (voluntary teaching, voluntary nonteaching, municipal teaching, municipal nonteaching or proprietary), service status (private or ward) and type of professional service (obstetrician, house staff or other physician). This study is an excellent illustration of the insights that can be gained by combining the three approaches to evaluation: structure, process and outcome. A more recent, and less ambitious, study of the same type is an analysis of postoperative mortality of pediatric surgery in a teaching hospital.[85] Both studies illustrate the magnitude of the problem of quality control. The perinatal mortality study showed that 42 percent of all perinatal deaths in mature infants had preventable factors associated with them. In 82 percent of preventable deaths there were errors of medical judgment. The study of postoperative mortality showed that such deaths occur in only 0.5 percent of pediatric operations. However, 90 percent of such deaths were considered preventable.

The final method of implementing end result assessment is through the design of *special studies,* which fall into that area of overlap between research, operational research, and program evaluation that has been identified in a previous section of this volume. Three such studies have been referred to already.[82, 84, 85] Others will be mentioned below.

Two kinds of end result studies may be distinguished according to method, provided one recognizes the occurrence of mixed or intermediate forms. The first may be called observational and the second, experimental.

OBSERVATIONAL STUDIES

Observational studies utilize well-established epidemiological methods to study relationships between outcome and existing modes of program organization.[86-88] The Kohl and Thompson studies are examples.[82, 84] Another is the study of perinatal mortality and prematurity among enrollees of the Health Insurance Plan of Greater New York as compared to the general New York City population.[89, 90] Other studies of this type include a study of case fatality in teaching and nonteaching hospitals and of client behavior and outcomes in Old Age Assistance recipients enrolled in a prepaid group practice, as compared with those receiving care from the traditional welfare sources.[91, 92] Such studies tend to be retrospective, but they could also be prospective. The essential distinguishing characteristic is not that they are retrospective or prospective in nature, but that the investigator has no control over the allocation of subjects to the medical care programs under study. Therefore, he must introduce control through the analysis of data in such a way that similar segments of the study populations are compared and/or differences related to population characteristics other than medical care are accounted for statistically. How far one goes in introducing such adjustments depends on what the investigator considers to be reasonable, and to what extent the generally limited sample can be divided into subgroups without running into the problem of small numbers. The major weakness of these studies is that no matter how carefully the data are handled the possibility of lack of comparability in populations remains. The conclusions are therefore never established beyond doubt. These difficulties notwithstanding, observational studies can provide essential insights into the implications of medical care organization and raise questions that can be definitively answered by more carefully controlled studies. Observational studies are often the only realistic method available to examine significant issues in the medical care field.

Experimental studies involve the introduction of planned change in the medical care system and the random allocation of persons to receive care from two or more alternative programs. The investigator thereby has considerable control over the situation and the design of the study. Also, the problem of bias arising from noncomparability of study and control populations, as encountered in observational studies, is dealt with more effectively. Consequently, there is much greater assurance that differences in end results are due to planned differences in the programs of care rather than in the persons seeking and receiving care. Examples of experimental studies of medical care organization that include end result measurement are a study of the effect of organized home care by Bakst and Marra,[93] a study of comprehensive outpatient care by Katz et al.[94] and a study of a new form of organizing welfare services in New York City.[95, 96]

Both observational and experimental studies may involve either comparisons of populations before and after the introduction of changes in the program or contemporaneous study of two or more programs.

The proper design of experimental and observational studies requires expert knowledge in sampling, research design and other fields of statistics. Two brief, but excellent, discussions are recommended to the beginner in this field. The first, by Elinson, is a general introduction to methods in sociomedical research.[97] The other, by Horvitz, deals with applications to program evaluation.[98] Further discussion of the case for end result studies, some brief descriptions of examples of such studies, and references to additional studies are to be found in the paper by Shapiro.[54] Leonard et al. also discuss the uses of the experimental approach in the evaluation of patient care.[99]

We might conclude with the observation by Shapiro that the circumstances now are more favorable than at any time in the past for conducting observational and experimental studies of the effect of organization on the process and end results of medical care. There has been considerable refinement in methods; basic data are more widely available and there are more opportunities to design, implement and evaluate organized programs under public and private auspices.[54]

Part III:

ISSUES OF METHOD AND TECHNIQUE

Some General Requirements

Rosenfeld has summarized as follows the general specifications for methods of quality appraisal:

> To be ideally suited as an instrument of program evaluation the method of measurement should be: (1) sufficiently sensitive to distinguish differences in the quality of care among units studied; (2) objective in that different observers would arrive at similar ranking of units with similar magnitudes of differences between them; (3) valid in that it would reflect the quality of service in terms of current concepts of good medical practice; (4) based on sufficiently general principles of medical practice to be applicable to the several specialties; and (5) practical of application at costs that are not prohibitive.[100]

He has identified, as well, several stages in the development of any system of measurement that are also applicable to the assessment of quality.

The first stage is recognition of a need for measurement and for instruments specially designed to accomplish that purpose. The second stage involves testing the values and limitations of the measurement tool by determining validity, reliability, sensitivity and costs. The third stage might be called "socialization" of the instrument: "the extension of its use, as a convenience, so that a common language is built up for communication and expression of observation." The final stage consists of continuing research to improve the instrument and adapt it to changing needs (Reference 6, pages 3–4).

In this section there will be a discussion of some technical issues that the administrator needs to understand no matter which of the approaches and methods, or combination thereof, described in previous sections he chooses in order to appraise the quality and use of service in his program.

Sources of Information

The essential first step to appraisal is <u>collection of information</u>. The kind of information available has a fundamental effect on what appraisal mechanisms are feasible or preferable, and on how reliable and valid are the judgments concerning care. In this section, the various sources of information usually available to the administrator will be reviewed and their use for quality appraisal evaluated.

Observation of practice would appear to be the most obvious and direct method of obtaining information for the assessment of care. It is likely to be an important source of information feeding into the informal system of colleague interaction and control that operates in any highly organized setting for the provision of care.* However, its use as the basis of a formal mechanism of control would seem to be confined to teaching students and training junior colleagues.

The direct observation of practice is almost the only way of evaluating the process of care in situations where medical records are unavailable or too inadequate to form a basis for judgment. Hence, it has been used to study the quality of general practice in this country and abroad.[11, 101, 102]

Direct observation has many limitations. The most important is that observation is likely to alter the practice of the physician who is being observed. Since the change is likely to be in the direction of better care, the assessment made is probably of the capacity to perform rather than of usual levels of performance. This objection has been countered by assurances that the physician under observation may be unaware of the true purpose of the study, that he becomes rapidly accustomed to the presence of the observer, and that he is unable to change confirmed habits of practice.

An additional limitation to the use of direct observation in studies of quality, whether administrative or research-oriented, is the great deal of professional time that it requires and, hence, its costliness.

Clinical records are the source documents for most studies of the medical care process. They are directly, or through the use of derivative abstracts, the basis for case review and for systems of statistical display and analysis. The availability and adequacy of the clinical record are therefore matters of central importance to quality assessment.

The availability of records is not always a matter within the control of the administrator. Access to office records of physicians, for example, is a rarity. For this reason, the use of records has been restricted to the assessment of care in hospitals, outpatient departments of hospitals, and prepaid group practice. When records are available, the major issue then becomes their adequacy as a basis for assessment, and the question most often asked is whether the assessment made is to be of the care actually provided or of the care imperfectly reflected in the written record. There are here two major problems: of completeness and of veracity.

The account of care inscribed in the hospital record may be incom-

---

* Freidson and Rhea have studied some of the avenues of, and obstacles to, the dessemination of information in medical care organizations.[103]

plete partly because care has been provided and procedures performed prior to hospital admission. Incompleteness in the record may result from inadequate recording of adequate care or from inadequacies in the care itself. The problem is to disentangle these several causes.

An area of special weakness is the frequent absence from the record of adequate data on the social and emotional factors related to illness and management. The record seldom provides information concerning patient satisfaction and the patient-physician relationship. Certain dimensions of the quality of care thus cannot be evaluated through the record.

Records of care in office practice, even when available, are notoriously incomplete and inadequate. Both Peterson and Clute have reported the prevailing inadequacies of recording in general practice.[11, 101] On the other hand, a recent study of the office practice of a sample of members of the New York Society of Internal Medicine suggests that abstracts of office records can be used to obtain reproducible judgments concerning the quality of care.[104] However, since this finding concerns a particular group of physicians who are more likely to keep good records than the average, it may not be applicable to the office practice of specialists in general. Moreover, for one reason or another, the original sample drawn for this study suffered a 61 percent attrition rate.

In addition to incompleteness in the record, there may be questions concerning the veracity of recorded statements. First, there may be inaccuracies in the recording of events that transpire during the course of care. Second, there may be errors in the data which the physician uses to arrive at a diagnosis and a plan of treatment, as pointed out in a previous section of this volume.

These errors in recording point up the need for corrective action. The fundamental approach to the problem of incompleteness is to improve records and recording. Comparative studies require completeness and uniformity in records as well as agreement on definitions and procedures. Ferber has made some recommendations concerning the definition and recording of primary and secondary diagnoses, complications, consultations, operative procedures, and so forth.[105] Improvements are especially needed in the records of ambulatory care.

It may be possible to expand the medical record to include more data on the social and psychological components of the management of illness and the interactional aspects of the patient-physician relationship. This may best be done through a systematic effort to include specific items of information in nurses' notes and social service records. These additional sources could then be used for the assessment of dimensions of quality not included in the usual appraisals of technical performance.[5]

Failing fundamental improvements in the quality of the record itself, the assessor has to resort to secondary measures to remedy the present incompleteness of many records of patient care. One approach is to choose for evaluation certain diagnostic categories which are likely to be supported by recorded evidence in addition to the physician's own entries.[38] This explains, in part, the frequent use of surgical operations as material for studies of quality. Lembcke has emphasized the need to assemble, and use in assessment, all collateral recorded evidence, including nurses' notes—partly to achieve greater completeness, and partly to check on veracity.[41] Other investigators have tried to compensate for incompleteness in the record by conducting supplementary interviews with the attending physician and making appropriate amendments.[12, 36, 37] Unfortunately, only one of these studies (length of stay in Michigan hospitals) contains a report of what difference such an additional step made. In this study "the additional medical information elicited by means of personal interviews with attending physicians was of sufficient importance in 12.6 percent of the total number of cases studied to warrant a reclassification of the evaluation of necessity for admission and/or length of stay."[106, 12] When information obtained by interview is used to correct or supplement the patient record, the assumption may have to be made that this additional information has equal or superior validity. Morehead, who has had considerable experience with this method, suggests that such an assumption may be unwarranted:

> The cases were discussed with the physician, who was given the opportunity to comment on each case and, in theory, supply missing information. This aspect of the study method was not felt by any of the surveyors to be of value. It invariably placed the physician being reviewed on the defensive and became an apology for his record keeping. It did not serve to elucidate further understanding of the clinical handling of the case—a very sensitive area when compared to that of record keeping. On the other hand, the group physicians frequently did not feel these discussions were thorough enough, particularly when they felt, as was generally the case, that a lowered score resulted from failure to give credit for items said to have been done whose results were remembered.[40]

In addition to checks on completeness, it may be necessary to check the veracity of the events described in the record. Lembcke did this by searching in the record, including the nurses' notes, for what appeared to be the most valid evidence of the true state of affairs.[41] We have already discussed the issues related to verifying the accuracy of the basic data, such as physical findings and diagnostic test results, which are used in patient management.

We began the discussion of the medical record as a source of information for the assessment of quality by asking whether the object was to evaluate the quality of the record or the quality of care that the record portrays, often imperfectly. The two may in fact be interrelated. Appropriate recording is itself an important dimension of the quality of care. It may be recalled that recording was a factor in two of the definitions of quality quoted in the introductory section (pages 8 and 9) of this volume. This is because the record is a major instrument of communication in the management of care and, as such, an indispensable tool whenever two or more persons must cooperate in the provision of care. It is a major vehicle for the coordination of care during any one episode, and for the continuity of care over time. For this and other reasons, the Joint Commission on Accreditation of Hospitals pays considerable attention to the components of the record, its proper maintenance, the administrative organization of the medical record department, and the professional surveillance and control of the recording function.[107]

Although a relationship between the quality of recording and the quality of care has been generally assumed, it has not been empirically confirmed. Most students of the field would agree that good recording is likely to be associated with good care mainly because the conditions that bring about good care are also responsible for bringing about good recording. It is also assumed that, if there are discrepancies, the care provided is probably better than the record would indicate. This may not be the case; and one should entertain the possibility that the record may present too rosy a picture of the actual events.

Using an ingenious method of analysis, Rosenfeld has shown that recording and quality of care are positively correlated.[100] He handled the problem of separating recording from care by examining the reasons for downrating the quality of care documented in each patient record which had been used for evaluating quality. He demonstrated that the quality of care was rated down partly because of what could have been poor recording ("presumptive evidence") and partly for reasons independent of recording ("substantial evidence"). He also found that individual hospitals tended to receive similar ratings on both of these criteria, indicating the correlation between quality of recording and quality of care. Clute, on the other hand, was able to evaluate the quality of care in general practice by direct observation, and to compare what he observed with the general practitioner's records. He concludes that ". . . the lack of adequate records is not incompatible with practice of a good, or even an excellent quality. . . ." Unfortunately, neither Clute nor Peterson *et al.* provides a statement of the correlation between the quality of the record and the quality of care as assessed by direct observation. Studies that permit this kind of comparison are needed to clarify the uses and limitations of the record in assessment.

A final limitation to the use of records is the possibility that the examiner will be biased by his knowledge of the identity of the physicians and/or the identity of the institution.[106] It is known that physicians tend to have fairly well-formed opinions on the reputations of physicians and hospitals, and sometimes act upon these in seeking care for themselves and members of their own families.[108-111] But there have been no studies to demonstrate the effect of personal opinions on the assessment of the quality of care based on record review. Such studies are needed. In the meantime, it would appear prudent to obscure, where possible, information that might permit the reviewer to identify the source of care.

A great deal of the preceding discussion on ways to handle problems of incompleteness, unveracity, and bias are most pertinent to research studies of the quality of care where it is necessary to arrive at some valid measure of quality. The administrative objective of record review may be different and, in a sense, less stringent. For administrative purposes, it may be sufficient to obtain evidence that something might be wrong in the course of management. Once errors are suspected, it would be mandatory to consult the physicians involved and there would be little interest in locating precisely a given episode of care on any sort of quantitative quality scale. Instead, it would be important to create a situation in which professionals can learn to improve the standards of care.

Knowledge of the identity of the physician or hospital may be of value where it is important to scrutinize with particular care practice known to have been deficient in the past. It would be prudent, however, to supplement this with "blind" reviews to make certain that the review mechanism is capable of dealing impartially with all.

These differences in the use of the record for assessment, resulting from the purpose of such assessment, are extremely important. They illustrate a general principle, the applicability of which will be demonstrated repeatedly in subsequent pages of this volume, that the demands made on the method of assessment must always be adjusted to the purposes of that assessment.

Record Abstracts are the more proximate sources of information for the systems of statistical display and analysis described earlier. Abstracts of medical records may also be prepared in advance, usually by nonphysicians, and may serve as a basis for case review. Needless to say, the abstracts reflect all the limitations of the original record but need not be discussed again. There are a number of additional considerations, pertaining specifically to the preparation and use of record abstracts, which will be explored in this section.

When record abstracts are used as a basis for statistical display and analysis, the first consideration is the amount of information to be assembled in the abstract. This, of course, depends upon the system's objectives and projected uses. We have already referred to the rather restricted emphasis on length of stay analysis in the Hospital Utilization Project (HUP), and the correspondingly sparse abstract.[30-32] Shindell has emphasized the need to limit abstracted information to meet the minimum objectives of the system and to what can be effectively used. A large amount of unused information may repel potential users and is costly. Moreover, error is more likely to occur, especially if abstracting involves a search through the medical record. Partly in order to minimize such errors, the HUP abstract limits information to that available on the face sheet of the medical record.[30]

In some respects, the HUP approach is in contrast with that used by the Commission on Professional Hospital Activities (CPHA). The CPHA abstract, as we have described, contains more information on more aspects of medical care. In fact, some feel that more, rather than less, is required for effective quality appraisal (Payne in Reference 6, page 143). Should additional information be needed, an arrangement for special studies can be made with CPHA to utilize the blank space that is provided on the abstract. The design of the abstract form is guided by the following requirements as described by Slee:

> (1) the traditional information needs of the hospital must be met; (2) the information carried should be relevant to assessment of the quality of care; (3) no new forms should be required of the physician; (4) the data should require no interpretation by the clerical personnel; and (5) completion time should not exceed perhaps five to seven minutes.[27]

The value of additional information to be gained by expansion of the abstract form must be weighed against the disadvantages of increased abstracting time, the additional cost and complexity of data processing and display, and the probability that the hospital and physicians will be overwhelmed with information they cannot use.[27a]

One method of introducing additional information is to use different abstract forms for different diagnostic conditions. Such a development would, however, pose severe problems in operating separate information systems for each class of patients, especially where any one patient might fall in more than one class.[27]

There are some questions concerning the accuracy of the abstracting process in systems such as those of HUP and CPHA. The record abstract is usually prepared by the hospital medical record librarian or under her direct supervision. Shindell and London report that experience in HUP has shown that "accuracy in coding is increased if responsibility for completing abstracts is given to a specific member of the medical records department rather than rotated among a number of persons."[31]

Quality control over the process of abstracting is an important matter. CPHA has instituted a number of activities to educate, train and supervise those persons involved in the use of their system in the participating hospitals.[28] This is in addition to quality control procedures within the central agency itself. Doyle has described the quality control procedures in HUP:

> When completed, the abstracts are submitted to the control unit of the project's data processing center at Blue Cross where they are checked for completeness and where all coding is verified. The output of each clerk is subject to a very tight quality control sampling inspection plan. Based on the results of this sample inspection the entire output is accepted or rejected. If rejected, the work is returned to the clerk for 100 percent verification. If acceptable, the abstracts are keypunched and verified into punch card form for machine processing. As the cards are being processed by the computer, the information undergoes a series of automatic checks to further insure the accuracy of the data. The computer is then used to assemble the data and print various listings (diagnosis and surgical). At the time of the study, the listings were being verified by personnel before being forwarded to the hospitals. Upon receipt at the hospital, the data were again subjected to inspection and all discrepancies were reported back to the data processing center for correction of data captured in punch card form for future statistical runs and analyses.[112]

Certain considerations pertain to the use of record abstracts as a basis for case review. A major advantage of using the record abstract for this purpose is that it may be prepared by a less skilled person, thereby allowing the hard-to-get expert to concentrate on the actual task of evaluation. However, unless rigid guidelines were formulated in advance to control it, abstracting would involve the exercise of judgment as to relevance and importance. For this reason, abstracts have been used only in those studies that have explicitly formulated standards: the "scientific" audits of Lembcke,[41-43] the "criteria approach" of Payne [44-47] and the exploratory study of the office practice of New York internists by the University of Pittsburgh group.[104] Morehead, who has a preference for case review using implicit criteria, has questioned the value of record abstracts in quality assessment. She summarizes her experience as follows:

> It was thought that perhaps a case summary prepared by a nurse would facilitate a surveyor's orientation, particularly in excessively large records. The consensus of the surveyors was that such summaries, regardless of how well prepared, tended to interpose a completed picture between the clinician and the record and influence his train of thought as he followed the progress of any given patient. There was very strong feeling on the part of all the physicians involved in these projects that only through a detailed personal review of an entire medical record could a judgment on the quality of care be made with assurance; nurses' notes, in particular, were of value. Therefore, regardless of the cumbersome nature of the process of obtaining photostatic copies of records in their entirety, and the additional time and money required, all surveyors felt that there was no place for non-physicians

in the preparation of material to be reviewed if the objective was to be the judgment of clinical performance.[40]

The difference of opinion between those who use record abstracts and those who do not probably rests on the distinction already made: the prior formulation of explicit standards and criteria.

Unfortunately, there is little published empirical evidence concerning the reliability and validity of abstracting itself and of quality judgments based on abstracts versus those based on review of the entire record. Kroeger *et al.* have reported a high level of agreement between physicians and highly trained nonphysicians abstracting the same office record. They have also studied the degree of agreement among several judges reviewing the same group of case abstracts. Out of 10 judges, who examined each of 21 abstracts and assigned them to one of four categories of quality, over half were in perfect agreement on the grade given in 13 of the 21 abstracts. It was felt that performance would have been improved if specific criteria for grading and scoring had been supplied.[104]

Health Insurance Claim Forms are seldom used for the full-fledged evaluation of quality. However, they are invariably subjected to clerical and professional verification and are sometimes used as a basis for more complex systems of utilization control.[17, 113]

The information on claim forms is, of necessity, rather limited. By comparing the information in the claim with that in abstracts of records, Doyle found that most items of information on the claim are quite accurate except for age, use of certain types of services and, most important, diagnosis. Discrepancies occurred in 25 percent of diagnoses. In seven percent of cases the diagnosis on the claim agreed with the admission diagnosis in the abstract, in eight percent with a secondary final diagnosis, and in 10 percent with none of the diagnoses in the abstract. Length of stay data were reasonably accurate, with length of stay derived from the claim tending to be, on the average, 0.3 days shorter. The conclusion to be drawn is that claims cannot be used for studies of length of stay by diagnosis without prior verification of the validity of the diagnosis given in the claim. Validity may vary by specific diagnosis, fineness of diagnostic categorization to be used in the analysis, and by hospital or health plan. Information on diagnosis could be obtained from some other more accurate source for use in conjunction with items of valid information in the claim.[112]

Reputations of physicians and hospitals may be one additional method of obtaining information concerning the quality of care. However, the information obtained is not in the form of data on the basis of which a judgment is made concerning quality, but is a finished judgment of quality.

Georgopoulos and Mann were able to rate and rank community hospitals using opinions concerning the medical care, and other characteristics, held by different categories of managerial, professional and technical persons working in, or connected with, each hospital, as well as opinions held by knowledgeable persons in the community. The responses were sufficiently consistent and discriminating to permit the hospitals to be ranked with an apparently satisfactory degree of reliability. The authors provide much evidence that the various opinions, separately held, were intercorrelated to a high degree. But they were not able to demonstrate that these judgments were valid by comparing them with truly external criteria of the quality of care.[108]

More recently, Denton et al. asked groups of knowledgeable physicians to judge the quality of care in the general hospitals in each of five cities. There was a high degree of concurrence among physicians in their judgments. A study of hospital characteristics showed that physician judgment was most highly correlated with hospital size and number and scale of residency training programs.[109] While these relationships appear reasonable, the less than significant correlation with medical school affiliation is difficult to reconcile with generally accepted assumptions and with the findings of studies, such as those of Morehead et al., that show the preeminence of medical school affiliated hospitals in rendering quality care.[38, 39]

Densen has recounted a personal experience that demonstrates the accuracy with which a particularly qualified physician can judge the effectiveness of care. A physician who had surveyed the care in medical groups in the Health Insurance Plan of Greater New York was able to predict with great accuracy the position, on a three-point scale, of that group in perinatal mortality. "There was a beautiful correlation between his rating and the perinatal mortality rates" (Reference 6, page 100).

Maloney et al. have reported that physicians, in choosing other physicians to provide care for themselves and members of their families, appear to use criteria generally accepted to be correlated with the quality of care. These include specialization and medical school affiliation. It was concluded that physician choice may be used as a method of identifying high quality care.[110] Bynder has reanalyzed the data of this study and concludes that physicians do indeed make such choices but that these are restricted to situations considered to be of serious import. In less serious situations, social factors become more important in determining the choice of the care-providing physician.[111]

It is not clear what use the administrator can make of reputational information in the conduct of his program. For one thing, the validity of the information is not well established. Such information

SAMPLING AND SELECTION

should be of some value in setting up a program and, particularly, in deciding on the sources which are to be favored in the purchase of care. However, reputational information is not readily applicable in a system of quality surveillance and, therefore, would be of peripheral relevance to the concerns of this volume. The creative administrator may, however, wish to speculate about the uses of the reputational approach to quality assessment.

Sampling and Selection

Universe to be Sampled. The first step in sampling is to specify precisely the universe to be sampled, and this choice in turn depends on what kind of generalizations one wishes to make. If the provider is to be the object of study, then one needs a sample of providers and of the care they furnish. If the object of study is the population, then one needs a sample of persons and of the care they receive, usually from a variety of sources. Whether providers or populations are the object of study depends on the general framework for quality appraisal which, as we have described in our introductory section, fixes the level and scope of concern for administrative activities as a whole.

Population samples make it possible to evaluate the total impact of a medical care system on the health-related behavior and health status of the population. As already described, end result evaluation is the most appropriate frame of reference for this purpose. Population samples also make it possible to tap certain aspects in the universe of care not readily available through sampling of the records of care received. Due to the manner in which such records are categorized by diagnosis and filed, it is difficult to identify elements, other than diagnostic categories, that require investigation and management. (It is not easy, for example, to identify cases of "headache" or "abdominal pain.") The records also give no information concerning situations in which care was not received, though it might have been required. Population studies make it possible to capture this missing component.

If the provider is to be studied, there is a further decision to make: is the objective of the study to obtain a representative picture of the care a provider or group of providers actually give? or is it to test the providers' general competence and their capacity to perform? A true picture of the care provided requires drawing probability samples of care, while the capacity to perform is tested through selective sampling.

Several factors enter into the selection of cases for testing the capacity of physicians to perform. The clinical situations chosen tend to be both demanding in terms of diagnostic and therapeutic acumen, and more significant in terms of the probable impact that mismanagement would have on the client. The situations should also be selected with an eye to whether their frequency in the provider's practice is of significance. Another important consideration is whether testing performance is relevant to the several dimensions of quality that one wishes to explore. Certain situations are more suitable for testing the technical dimensions of care, whereas others might offer more discrimination in testing the nontechnical dimensions. The choice of situation is also dependent, as we shall see, on the degree to which standards of management are clearly formulated and agreed upon within the profession. A final factor is the degree to which valid and complete information concerning the situation under study may be found in the medical record.

The relevance of these several considerations to the selection of cases for assessment is clearly illustrated in the following account that describes the procedure in studies of ambulatory care in the Health Insurance Plan of Greater New York:

> Obviously, the way in which the ten cases of illness were selected for review was a crucial point in the study design. It was agreed that no purpose would be served by a random selection of cases, because either the majority of patients coming to the family physicians had conditions that were of a self-limiting nature or sufficient documentary evidence for supporting the diagnosis would not be available. The decision was made that cases would be restricted to specific major illnesses where confirmatory evidence would be expected.... Diabetes, hypertension, coronary artery disease, peptic ulcer, anemia and kidney disease were the conditions selected for review in medicine. Cases of carcinoma and liver disease were included when encountered. It was felt that these cases would need fairly extensive diagnostic procedures, [would] involve the group specialists and facilities, and would require the physician to exercise more skill and acumen than are required by more common conditions such as respiratory infections and minor trauma. An attempt was made to select two cases from each disease category mentioned in order to obtain a broad picture of physician performance.[40]

What consequences does the selection of cases for review have on the results obtained and their interpretation? The answer is to be found in the extent of homogeneity within medical practice.

Homogeneity and Heterogeneity. We have already discussed, in the introductory section to this volume, some issues of homogeneity and heterogeneity in the quality of care. We described the many dimensions of the quality of care and spoke of the possibility that the performance of an individual physician might not be at a uniform level with respect to all dimensions. It is also likely that the practice of any one physician, or institution, will vary with respect to any one dimension. For example, the physician may perform better, within any one technical dimension, for certain diseases than for others. This

HOMOGENEITY

may be unrelated to technical difficulty and reflect, instead, special interest, aptitude, knowledge or training. In addition to variability *within* physicians and institutions, there is likely to be variability *among* physicians and institutions. Knowledge of the nature and magnitude of variability is essential for devising efficient sampling procedures.

The empirical evidence concerning homogeneity and heterogeneity is not extensive. Both the Peterson and Clute studies of general practice showed a high degree of correlation between performance of physicians in different components or dimensions of care (history, physical examination, treatment, and so forth).[11, 101] Morehead reports that in the HIP studies of ambulatory care there was consistency in the performance of each physician with respect to the entire group of his cases, which were selected in the manner already described above:

> Considerable consistency was noted in the ratings of individual cases of physicians in the various categories; e.g., a physician in the 2nd rating class usually had the majority of his cases scored between 61 and 75.[40]

Rosenfeld demonstrated that the differences in quality ratings among several diagnoses selected within each area of practice (medicine, surgery and obstetrics-gynecology) were not large. Although the differences among hospitals by area of practice appeared by inspection to be larger, they were not large enough to alter the rankings of the three hospitals studied.[100] Morehead has reported that the performance of physicians within each medical group in the Health Insurance Plan of Greater New York tended to be homogeneous. "Birds of a feather flock together" (Reference 6, page 65). If such findings are sustained, it would be reasonable to proceed on the assumption that evaluation of a well-selected number of cases will give a true picture of a physician's, or institution's, general capacity to perform.

There are other studies, however, that show a significant degree of heterogeneity and indicate that the "diagnostic mix" of the cases selected for evaluation can influence the results. This is illustrated through a comparison of the findings from the two studies of the quality of care received by Teamster families in New York City. In the first study, selected hospitalized diagnoses were evaluated.[38] In the second study, a random sample of all hospitalizations were evaluated.[39] "The very fact that the patient was in hospital took him out of the minor illness category, a category deliberately avoided in the HIP studies of ambulatory care." [40] Interestingly enough, the two studies arrived at almost identical proportions of "optimal" and "less than optimal" care for the entire populations studied. This must have been coincidental, since the percent of optimal care, in the second study, varied greatly by diagnostic category, from 31 percent for medicine to 100 percent for ophthalmology (nine cases only). If such variability exists, the "diagnostic mix" of the sample of care must be a matter of considerable importance in assessment. In comparing the second Teamster study to the first, differences in "diagnostic mix" were thought to have resulted in lower ratings for medicine and higher ratings for obstetrics-gynecology. "The most probable explanation for the ratings in medicine being lower in the present [second] study is the nature of the cases reviewed." The factor responsible is less ability to handle illness "which did not fall into a well recognized pattern." For obstetrics and gynecology the finding of the second study ". . . differed in one major respect from the first study, where serious questions were raised about the management of far more patients. The earlier study consisted primarily of major abdominal surgery, whereas the later randomly selected group contained few such cases and had more patients with minor conditions." [39] To recapitulate, as opposed to evaluating only selected diagnoses, taking a mixed bag of all hospital cases resulted in a *lower* estimate of quality in medicine and a *higher* estimate of quality in obstetrics and gynecology. The occurrence of changes in opposite directions as a result of one change in sampling shows how complex is the phenomenon under investigation, and points to the need for much further study.

Some of the findings of the Teamster studies may be explained by the many causes of variability in quality of care received by a population group. Variability results partly from differences in the performance of the same physician in certain diagnostic categories as compared to others, and partly because other physicians are called upon to provide care for different diagnoses or situations of varying complexity and seriousness. For example, all nine cases of eye disease received optimal care because "this is a highly specialized area, where physicians not trained in this field rarely venture to perform procedures." [39] The actual allocation of medical care functions is, of course, a distinctive feature of each medical care system, and would vary from place to place.

Morehead has reported another instance in which the method of sampling has significant consequences for the findings. What was revealed was variability in the performance of a given institution with respect to different dimensions of quality:

> During the period of the HIP studies, one of the very strong hospitals in the City requested that a review be made of the records in their medical outpatient department by the same technique. After a review of some 40 cases selected from the medical department's file, it was felt that the study was of

little value in terms of ultimate recommendations; not one case received less than the allocated 100 points. Almost as an afterthought, a second review was instituted: this time cases were selected at random from the admitting office of the outpatient department. This one change gave a considerably different picture of patient care. A major weakness was shown to exist by the lack of coordination between specialty departments. For example, a woman was followed for more than 6 years by the opthalmology department where she went frequently for new glasses. Funduscopic reports over the years showed increasing evidence of degenerative changes and vascular disease. However, it was not until the sixth year, when the woman suffered a stroke, that she came to the attention of the medical department.[40]

No better example can be found of the multidimensionality of quality and the heterogeneity of practice, and of their implications to sampling in the assessment of quality.

Sampling in Administrative Surveillance. Under the rubric of "sampling," we have so far discussed some general issues of particular relevance to quality assessments with a research orientation. The purpose of such assessments is to obtain a representative picture of quality in relation to some defined universe, a purpose which may be equally applicable to certain objectives of administrative surveillance. What is important is that under a different set of assumptions the administrator may find that a representative picture is irrelevant. When administrative appraisal seeks to obtain a true picture of care so that the nature and extent of deficiencies may be identified and corrective action planned, a representative sample of care obviously is needed. However, administrative effort may, after initial assessment, be directed at areas of particular weakness for purposes of detection, deterrence and education. What is then sought is a sample most sensitive to, and representative of, poor care. Samples for this purpose may be stratified, by disease or service, and weighted to correspond to the importance of the problem areas involved. Such samples will be less efficient for reviewing the whole pattern, but may be more efficient at detecting difficulties and maintaining surveillance over them.

Whether the primary objective is deterrence or education may, in itself, have an influence on the method of case selection. Presumably, deterrence would require more comprehensive coverage, and selection might thus include at least some cases from the practice of each physician on a hospital staff. Alternatively, there would have to be repeated sampling with a reasonably high likelihood of including any one physician or type of care. These considerations are analogous to the duality of emphasis on individual wrongdoing versus the identification of patterns of care which we have already described in a previous section.

The issue of yield, in terms of erroneous practices discovered, is very important to quality assessment within the administrative framework. The case review of large numbers of acceptable cases is costly and not educationally rewarding. Also, the members of the staff conducting the review may lose interest if "positive" findings are few and far between.

The field of industrial quality control has developed methods of sampling and analysis that take into account specified tolerances concerning detection and nondetection of error. Moroney gives a brief description of such methods.[114] A more detailed discussion may be found in a more recent monograph by Fetter.[115] For some reason, there has been little systematic exploration of the applicability of these concepts and techniques to the appraisal of the quality of medical care. Such work is, however, known to be currently in progress.[180a]

Sampling in Statistical Analysis and Display Systems. Generally these have been based on total samples of the care provided in any given institution. In part, this has been due to other uses of the data which require total coverage—accounting and the maintenance of indexed diagnostic and operative files required by accrediting organizations. When there is no reason to account for, or list, all cases, the advantages of sampling should be seriously considered.

Sampling in Case Reviews. The general considerations with regard to representativeness, scope of coverage and yield are fully applicable to the selection of cases for review. As already emphasized, there are almost no rigorous conceptual and methodological studies of sampling schemes for this purpose. The following account is, therefore, largely a description of current practice, with some attempt at evaluation.

The random sampling methods used in case selection, as Wolfe has pointed out, are usually of the systematic type. Typical schemes are selecting every nth case, for example every 10th, or choosing so many consecutive cases, for instance the first 50 cases beginning on a given date.[116] Shindell and London suggest the following method of selection for the case review phase of HUP:

> The medical record librarian would select a predetermined number of the most recently discharged patients with the primary diagnosis to be studied, going backwards from a recent date on which it is reasonable to assume most records are complete. The librarian will establish, to the best of her ability, that the diagnosis on the selected charts is the primary diagnosis under study and that it was responsible for the admission.
>
> Alternatively, one might select all cases discharged within a specific period of time, or use some random or systematic sampling technique which insures representativeness of a manageable number of cases. The suggestion that a consecutive series of most recent cases be utilized is based on the ease with

CASE REVIEWS

which these may be obtained from the monthly listings of cases produced by the data processing [system].[31]

The California Medical Association recommends the following procedure of case selection for utilization review:

> At the end of each month, the listings of all cases broken down by ICDA (International Classification of Diseases, Adapted) diagnostic category and by physician are inspected, with cases selected for review in the following manner:
>
> 1. When an individual physician has treated only one specific disease during the course of one month, this case will be reviewed. However, when more than one such diagnosis is treated by any one physician, *all* such cases are to be arrayed by date of hospital admission. The following sample design will then apply.
> 2. Where two, three, or four cases of the same diagnosis have been treated by the same physician, the *second* chronologically-ordered case will be selected.
> 3. Where five through nine such cases have been treated, the *first* and *fifth* chronologically-ordered cases will be selected.
> 4. Where ten through 19 cases have been treated, the *second, sixth* and *tenth* ordered cases will be selected for review.
> 5. Where 20 or more cases have been treated, select the *third, eighth, fourteenth* and *nineteenth* cases.[117]

The second approach to case selection is to choose certain categories of cases that are likely to be most revealing or productive in terms of the detection and correction of error, or in terms of some other defined objective. In utilization and quality review, the following types of cases have been considered to yield a higher proportion of improper use of hospital services.

1. *Long stay cases*—The reader is referred to the section on utilization control through certification for a discussion of what interval or intervals might be suitable to define a "long stay" case for purposes of review. The agencies involved in the Hospital Utilization Project (HUP) recommend that long stay be defined not as a single arbitrary period, but differently for each diagnosis. In their opinion:

> Experience has shown ... that reviewing cases of patients staying in a hospital beyond an arbitrary number of days is not likely to be productive unless the review is conducted for specific diagnostic groups. A study of eight-day maternity cases may be much more significant than an automatic study of all cases where the stay is thirty days or longer. This is not to say that long-stay cases may not represent complex socioeconomic problems which will require attention, and a study to determine possible difficulties in transferring persons in need of chronic care would certainly be productive and worthwhile. It is suggested, however, that concentration on long-stay cases on the part of a utilization committee will be more productive in saving days of care if "long-stay" becomes a meaningful term with respect to the individual diagnosis.[118]

The Length of Stay Package of the Commission on Professional and Hospital Activities (CPHA) lists individually as long stay cases all those that are discharged after the day on which falls the 90th percentile of that class of patients.[27a]

2. *Short stay cases*—

Over ten percent of all cases admitted to general hospitals are discharged after one or two days. Included among these cases may be a significant number admitted for diagnosis or minor surgery which might have been provided as effectively without admission. Each short-term case where the need for admission is questionable should be reviewed.[118]

The Length of Stay Package of CPHA lists individually as short-stay cases all those that are discharged before the day on which the 5th percentile of that class of patients falls. According to Slee, such cases are more likely to reflect questionable practice than do the long-stay cases as defined by CPHA (see above). Such short-stay cases "do not tend to be diagnostic admissions but rather patients who it would seem should have had a longer hospitalization—or none at all." [27a]

3. *Emergency admissions*—A sample of "emergency" admissions may be reviewed in order to verify the alleged need for priority to hospital admission. During periods of bed shortage and waiting lists, cases may be reviewed soon after admission as a method of concurrent control to assure the best allocation of a scarce resource.[118]

4. *Symptom diagnoses*—The presumption is that such cases have not been well studied prior to admission to hospital.

5. *Certain diagnostic categories, operations and other diagnostic or therapeutic procedures*—These are selected on the assumption that improper use or improper management are frequent. Over a number of years, the Commission on Professional and Hospital Activities has directed special attention, sometimes involving repeated studies and reports, to the following:

—**diseases:** acute coronary occlusion, stroke, toxemia of pregnancy, adult pneumonia, staphylococcal infection in pediatrics, diabetes, bleeding duodenal ulcer, acute infant diarrhea.
—**operations:** tonsillectomy, primary appendectomy, radical mastectomy, hysterectomy, tubal ligation, uterine suspension, lysis of abdominal adhesions.
—**procedures:** blood transfusions, use of antibiotics, use of anticoagulants.

The Pennsylvania Blue Cross has studied hysterectomies performed on women under 30 years old and prostatectomies performed on men under 30. They have also pointed to abuse in procedures such as proctosigmoidoscopies, arthrocenteses and basal metabolism determinations (which turned out to be photomotograms).[119]

6. *Unfavorable outcomes in which there might be preventability factors*—We have already commented on studies of adverse outcomes in the evaluation of the quality of care. These include case fatality, perinatal mortality, postoperative mortality, other postoperative complications, lacerations at delivery, transfusion reactions and other adverse reactions to therapy.

7. *Potentially preventable conditions*—Weinerman has pointed out that the hospital care of potentially preventable conditions provides a clue to the adequacy of care prior to hospitalization (Reference 6, page 44). Rheumatic heart disease in a young person would be an example. Certain complications of pregnancy and in the newborn would also qualify. Where the nature of the program permits it, the retrospective extension of case review into the prehospital period would be highly indicated.

8. *Providers under surveillance*—Certain physicians or hospitals, or certain categories of these, may have been designated for special intensive surveillance because of a record of previous improper use of services or the provision of inadequate care.

9. *Certain client behaviors*—Complaints by patients are always a signal for careful case review. If it is desired to extend the definition of quality, as one should, to embrace nontechnical dimensions of care, other client behaviors might also be cues for intensive analysis. Noncompliance with physician recommendations, such as leaving the hospital against advice, would be one such event.

A third approach to the selection of cases for review is to examine all, or samples of all, cases identified as aberrant or deviant by some other component of the system of utilization and quality control. We have already referred to the need to verify by review cases that have been certified to stay in the hospital beyond specified periods of time. This is an integral part of the system of Approval by Individual Diagnosis (AID) which has been described in a previous section. It constitutes the linkage of case review with a system of certification of hospital stay. Similarly, case review may be linked with a system of statistical review; the method of sampling of cases in one such system, the Hospital Utilization Project (HUP), was described above. There is another method of linkage which focuses on cases which are aberrant or deviant in a statistical sense. We have already described the manner in which a statistical system identifies such cases. It is possible to identify cases that deviate in terms of ranges and percentiles, or standard deviations from the mean. It is further possible to introduce, as we have described, corrections for differences in several characteristics that include diagnosis, age, whether an operation has been performed, and whether there is a secondary diagnosis.[29, 34] Wolfe has described in detail the development of a statistical screening system of this type for one diagnostic category: operations on the bilary tract.[116] Using regression analysis, Wolfe was able to reduce 355 variables considered likely to influence length of stay for this condition to five which explained 80 percent of the variation in length of stay. These were number of consultations, identity of the hospital, age, number of diagnoses during stay, and whether incision of the bile duct was or was not done. Using these control variables, the computer can identify cases that fall outside the expected length of stay. It is possible in each case to determine the mean length of stay and to set confidence limits. The strictness of the confidence limits determines the number of cases identified as "questionable" and designated for further case review. In the example described by Wolfe the results were as follows:

Tabulation III-1.

Confidence Limits	Questionable Cases (N=841)	
	Number	Percent
95%	5	0.6
87%	23	3.0
68%	66	7.0

By using Wolfe's system, one could adjust the sample size according to the degree of doubt about length of stay and depending on the resources available for carrying out case review. If it is desirable to reduce case review work to a minimum, one selects only cases in which the likelihood of inappropriate stay is very high (95 percent confidence limits). On the other hand, if one has the resources, and is unwilling to let cases go by even if there is reasonable doubt about length of stay, one chooses a lower confidence limit (68 percent). It is to be noted, however, that the case review load increases very rapidly.

The claims review procedures of a health insurance agency may be considered as part of the utilization control process. Cases that are questioned by this process, or are refused payment, constitute another group of "high risk" cases that are subjected to case review.

Sampling Variability. A specifiable error is attached to values (for example, means or proportions) derived from probability samples. The magnitude of the error depends on the variability of the measured phenomenon in the universe from which the sample was drawn and on the size of the sample. Consequently, one must consider whether, in comparing the average or percentage value in a sample of cases cared for by one provider with a sample of cases cared for by another, the observed differences could have arisen easily through chance or would be very unlikely to have occurred by chance. In other words, a statement needs to be made concerning statistical significance. A similar statement is needed to compare findings before and after the introduction of some control procedure or other change in the organization of medical care.

As methods of statistical appraisal become more highly developed, attention is increasingly directed toward providing estimates of sampling error and statements concerning the significance of observed differences. We have already mentioned that the "Length of Stay Package" developed by the Commission on Professional and Hospital Activities includes a statement of whether the average length of stay for any given category of cases in a participating hospital is or is not significantly different from the average length of stay for a large group of similar cases used as a standard for comparison.[28, 29] The Commission has also published 95 percent confidence limits for proportions or percentages. Upper and lower limits are easily read off a table given the numerator and denominator that constitute the ratio.[120]

Wolfe has described a method of case selection in which confidence limits are computed and the number of cases to be reviewed is adjusted correspondingly—another application of the statistical methods developed to deal with sampling variability.[116]

Sahai and Veney used data from the New Jersey Blue Cross plan for 1965 to compute and report sample sizes necessary to make certain estimates of length of stay by diagnostic category and by two age groups (under 65 and 65 and over) with specified precision and degree of confidence.[121] Of course these figures are applicable only when a random sample of all cases in a given category of cases has been selected.

Standards

Standards are an essential ingredient of any system of measurement or appraisal. In previous sections there were brief references to certain aspects of standards applicable to the assessment of the quality of medical care and the appropriateness of the use of health services. In this section there will be a more detailed description of nine aspects of these standards; source, validity, consensus, stability, transferability, configuration, level of stringency, explicitness and content.

Source. Standards of medical care may be said to derive from two sources: the opinions of health professionals and the actual practice of such professionals. The first of these may be called "normative" standards and the second "empirical" standards.

Normative standards are ideally derived from the opinions of what constitutes good practice as formulated by recognized and legitimate leaders in their respective professions. They may, however, be set by lesser experts, or represent values held generally by the rank and file.

A number of methods for setting or deriving normative standards may be used in studies of medical care quality. Lembcke relied on textbooks and standard publications.[41] Slee's belief was that textbook standards should be the basis for evaluating observed practice.[27] Expert panels drawn from the medical schools and the general medical community were used by the Michigan study of hospital utilization,[12] and by Payne in developing standards for his "criteria approach."[47] Morehead relied on the internalized standards of highly qualified practitioners, generally with a medical school appointment, who served as judges.[38-40] In the Rosenfeld study of the quality of hospital care, standards were formulated jointly by the research staff and qualified practitioners acting as consultants.[100] The normative standards of length of hospital stay by diagnostic category, which form the basis of the AID system of certification, were derived from polls of the staffs of participating hospitals.[23]

Perhaps the most ambitious undertaking in the development of normative standards was the formulation by Lee and Jones of what they called "The Fundamentals of Good Medical Care."[8] The opinions and records of 125 physicians were used, in part, to develop lists of the nature and amount of care needed for the "good" management of the whole range of disease categories. Given these standards, and information on the occurrence of illness, it was possible to estimate the resources and personnel needed to provide "good" medical care for the entire population. The following excerpt will help the reader obtain some appreciation of the nature and scope of this monumental work (Reference 8, page 156):

* * *

4. Pneumonia

General Practitioner—All pneumonia cases require medical care for a period of 2 days to 10 weeks, the average disability period being 42 days. The average number of visits per case is 15. Of these visits, 90 percent are in the home and 10 per cent are in the hospital. Each visit is of 25 minutes' duration.

Specialist—Fifteen cases, on an average, require consultation with an internist. These visits are of 15 minutes' duration, with 90 percent in the home and 10 per cent in the hospital.

Other Units of Service—Most cases need one nurse, and a certain proportion of cases need 2 nurses, for varying lengths of time. The average number of nursing days per case is 9. After the nurse has left, the average case requires the services of a full-time attendant for 5 days, and a part-time attendant for 7 days. Hospitalization for an average period of 3 weeks is required for

SOURCE

20 cases. All cases require one or more leucocyte counts and urinalyses, and one spinal puncture is indicated. A few X-ray examinations are necessary.

Physicians' Time

	Cases	Visits per Case	Total Visits	Minutes per Visit	Total Hours
General practitioner	100	15	1,500	25	625.00
Consultant [a]	15	1	15	15	3.75

Nursing Days

85 cases require 1 nurse for 7 days = 595 days
15 cases require 2 nurses for 10 days = 300 days

100 cases require a total of 895 days

Hospital Days

20 cases require an average of 21 days each = 420 days

Full-Time Attendant Days

100 cases require an average of 5 days each = 500 days

Part-Time Attendant Days

100 cases require an average of 7 days each = 700 days

Number of Laboratory Procedures

White blood count 250   Spinal puncture 1
Urinalysis 250

Number of X-Ray Examinations

Chest 10

[a] Internist.

* * *

These studies make it clear that normative standards are almost always not representative of professional opinion in any statistical sense. Their distinctive characteristic is that they rest on institutionalized notions of what is good practice. The derivation of the AID length of stay standards constitutes the nearest approach to formulation based on representative opinion. However, the attempt to do so did not fully succeed because out of 100 hospitals queried only 39 responded (Mikelbank in Reference 25, page 70).

Some of the uses and limitations of normative standards and several of their characteristics will be described in succeeding portions of this section.

By contrast with normative standards, empirical standards derive not from opinions, notions or pronouncements of what is good, but from actual practice. The practice may be that of leading professionals or of an outstanding teaching hospital affiliated with a medical school. These unusually qualified providers of care serve as a criterion. More usually, empirical standards are derived from practice in a general community, in which case they are often expressed in terms of distributions, averages, ranges and other measures of variability around an average value.

Empirical standards have several advantages. The first of these is realism and credibility. Actual practice is evidence that a given standard of care is not a visionary goal but a concrete reality that can be attained. By virtue of this, it gains in persuasiveness and acceptability. Shindell has emphasized how unimpressed hospital staffs are with length of stay standards formulated normatively by expert panels. By contrast, the impact of observing actual examples of lowered lengths of stay without apparent adverse effect in the same community is very great indeed.[30]

Another use of empirical standards is testing and modifying normative pronouncements in ways that shall be discussed below.

In situations where normative standards are poorly formulated and not readily codified, standards must be derived empirically. We have already referred to the paucity of quantitatively expressed normative criteria of end results, and suggested that this lack creates the necessity for empirical comparisons in end result assessment. There is reason to believe that to some extent the same is true for length of stay criteria. Furstenberg *et al.* used patterns of prescribing in medical care clinics and outpatient departments of hospitals as the standard to judge prescribing in private practice. This was because normative judgments concerning appropriate prescribing were not readily available.[122]

Empirical standards have a major limitation. Average practice cannot be accepted as a criterion of goodness unless a comparison is made with what is possible under the best circumstances. Even practice under optimal conditions must be judged by the normatively defined standard of excellence, which must remain the ultimate goal.

It is useful to examine, as we have done, the differences between normatively and empirically derived standards. It is equally important to be aware of the areas of interaction and overlap between them. Normative judgments underlie all standards no matter what their source. Empirical observations serve as standards only when a normative element of judgment is added. An example would be the declaration that average practice, or the top 5 percent in a distribution of an element of practice, is "good" or "acceptable." The distinction between normative and empirical standards becomes particularly ambiguous when a criterion institution is used as a standard of comparison. The criterion institution is chosen in the belief that its actual practice closely approximates what is taught to be the best practice. Lembcke used experience in the best hospitals to derive a corrective factor that softens the excessive rigidity of his normative standards. The corrective factor, expressed in terms of an acceptable percent of compliance with the standard, was designed to take account of contingencies not foreseen in the standards themselves. It also has the effect of being more realistically permissive because the correction factor is likely to be made up partly of acceptable departures from the norm and partly of unacceptable deviations from it.[41]

There is a remarkable paucity of studies that explore in a systematic way the relationships between normative and empirical standards. Mikelbank reports that the length of stay standards adopted for AID were generally above the average derived from practice in New Jersey hospitals. This is not surprising, since the physicians surveyed by Blue Cross were asked to give, for each diagnosis, an opinion on the "permissible maximum stay, without complication, [so that] the physician would be able to inform each patient as to the expected maximum duration of hospitalization benefits."[180a] It is difficult to say on what basis the responding physicians arrived at their estimates, but subsequent experience showed that the normative standards were the same as the observed mean in 105 diagnostic categories, 1–14 days in excess of the observed mean in 174 categories, and 1–6 days less than the observed mean in 36 categories.[23] Mikelbank has also provided data that indicate what the differences between the normative standards and actual practice signify in terms of hospital days actually used by the New Jersey population. During the first year following the institution of AID the aggregate hospital days actually used were only 82 percent of the days that would have been used had each case used the number of days allowed in the AID standards. During the twelve-month period prior to AID the hospital days actually used were 88 percent of those potentially allowed under AID standards. This suggests that AID had some success in reducing length of stay, and that standards of maximum allowable length of stay do not necessarily become minimum standards of stay.[23a] It would be useful to extend such comparisons to explore the relationship between the opinions of individual physicians concerning what is appropriate or good care and the actual practice of these same physicians.

Validity. The validity of almost all standards, whether normative or empirical, must ultimately derive from their demonstrated relationship to valued outcomes. Standards vary greatly in the degree to which this condition has been met. As Slee has pointed out, the validation of standards is generally in the province of medical research rather than quality assessment.[27] However, the student of quality must clearly distinguish standards that are extensively validated from those that rest on untested, though reasonable, assumptions. The assumptions themselves need to be clearly and explicitly recognized (Mindel Sheps in Reference 6, page 84). Some authorities in the field go further, and argue that agencies involved in the provision of care and the evaluation of their own services should plan to validate the standards that they use in their assessments (Densen in Reference 6, page 93).

In some situations, comparative studies of actual practice provide a test of validity. We have already referred to changes in length of stay standards based on observations that length of stay in some hospitals has been reduced without apparent adverse effect. Practice in a criterion institution can in this way challenge normatively derived standards.

Consensus. A certain degree of agreement among recognized leaders in the profession is necessary to permit convincing evaluation. Those aspects of care over which there is no wide agreement are therefore avoided in the selection of situations for assessment. A good example is the notable absence of tonsillectomies from the list of common operations frequently selected for surgical audit. The differences of opinion concerning the indications for tonsillectomy have led to the formulation of two sets of criteria representing the views of a pediatric panel and of an otolaryngology panel (Reference 47, page 48). Mikelbank reports that physician opinion concerning the permissible length of hospital stay for bronchopneumonia ranged from seven to 21 days. The distribution had two modes, one at 10 days and one at 14. When physician opinions were compared with actual practice, it was found that more than a third of cases stayed in hospital for longer than the 10-day mode, and about a fifth stayed for longer than the 14-day mode. The wide range in opinions, and the possible bimodality, show lack of agreement on permissible length of stay and/or considerable heterogeneity in the basic phenomenon (bronchopneumonia).[23]

Densen has pointed out that, in the development of standards, lack of agreement can be as important and revealing as agreement. The further investigation of those areas on which agreement cannot be obtained may be a productive area for research (Reference 6, page 24).

Stability. The validity of almost all standards of medical care is temporary and conditional. The standards are redefined as medical science and technology change. They are also influenced by changes in the organization of medical care services and by social developments that affect values and expectations relevant to medical care. For these reasons standards, especially those that are normatively defined, need to be constantly reformulated.

Rosenfeld has pointed out that reformulation can be brought about automatically if one bases quality judgments on patterns of care in a criterion institution, such as a teaching hospital, that is expected to keep alert to technical change:

> Use of the teaching hospital as a control provides the element of flexibility needed to adjust to the constantly changing scientific basis of the practice of medicine. No written standards, no matter how carefully drawn, would be adequate in five years.[100]

However, changes in social values and expectations may not be adequately reflected even in the practice of a teaching institution.

Transferability. Questions have been raised concerning the applicability to all groups and settings of standards formulated by one group or in one setting. There has been particular dissatisfaction with the application to general practice of standards and criteria elaborated by specialists who practice in academic settings. The major studies of general practice have made allowances for this.[11, 101] Little is known, however, about the strategies of "good" general practice and the extent to which they are similar to, or different from, the strategies of specialized practice in academic settings.

There are also differences of opinion concerning the applicability of externally derived or general standards to internal use by a hospital or to local use within a medical community. Is there, indeed, a definable community within which legitimate comparisons may be made? Payne emphasizes that the criteria for care set by external panels are only points of departure for consideration and, if need be, modification by each hospital staff.[47] Shindell points out the absence of generalizable standards of length of stay and emphasizes the importance of local practice, or the intrainstitutional "subculture," in determining what is acceptable.[30] Other students of the field tend to take a more universal view, pointing out that the normative standards of good practice, insofar as they represent what current medical science can achieve, should be of general applicability. However, there is room for legitimate variability when normative standards are either incompletely validated or not fully agreed upon.

Reasons for legitimate deviation from normative standards may also be found in the particular characteristics of medical care in a given locality. Local medical resources certainly place a limit on what may be realistically expected. Hospital use and length of stay, for example, would appropriately reflect the number and/or spatial distribution of physicians and population in a given locality.[123, 124] The availability of alternatives to hospitalization—outpatient diagnostic services and posthospital home care or extended facility care—would also influence standards of what is appropriate hospital use in a given community (Rosenfeld in Reference 25, page 113).

Configuration. It is useful to distinguish two kinds of phenomena or characteristics to which standards are applicable: "monotonic" and "inflected." Monotonic phenomena or characteristics are those about which one can say, "The more the better," or alternatively, "The less the better." It is obvious, for example, that the lowest possible mortality rate defines what is best with respect to mortality and survival. Similarly, it may be asserted that 100 percent of cases of diagnosed myocardial infarction should have had an electrocardiogram in the process of investigation. With respect to monotonic phenomena, the direction of movement that determines goodness is normatively defined. The difficulty is in establishing the degree of attainment of the goal under the best conditions of care. Since this is often not possible to fix with any degree of precision, one uses comparative studies and concludes that the program most closely approaching the goal has the highest level of care.

Inflected phenomena are more complex. They have an optimum value or range. Below and above this value, or range of values, quality is said to decrease. Slee suggests that the optimal range for pathologically positive tissue in primary appendectomy may be 80 to 90 percent. A percentage lower than this may mean too great a readiness to operate; a higher percentage may mean excessive conservatism and the possibility that inflamed appendices are allowed to go untreated. The problem with inflected phenomena is that the optimal values cannot be stated a priori, but must be determined empirically. As Mindel Sheps has pointed out, the necessity for empirical determination introduces significant limitations in the use of such phenomena as indicators of the quality of care.[9] Some of the problems of length-of-stay assessment arise because length of stay is an inflected phenomenon in which both overstay and understay indicate inappropriate use.

Level of stringency. The description of normative and empirical standards may have suggested to the reader that the former tend to be more stringent than the latter. While this is generally true, it is not so in all cases. Normative standards can be set at a variety of levels and so can empirical standards, depending on what type of practice is used as the criterion.

One factor to consider in deciding how stringent to make a standard is its ability to discriminate. Another factor is the yield of the standard, or the volume of aberrant cases identified in relation to the effort expended in reviewing cases.

With respect to the ability to discriminate, the standard may be so strict that no practice in real life can meet it. For example, Peterson and Barsamian report that although spermatic fluid examination of the husband should precede surgery for the Stein-Leventhal syndrome,

EXPLICITNESS

not one instance of such examination was noted, and this requirement had to be dropped from the criteria for assessment.[125] At the other extreme, in the study of general practice reported by Clute, blood pressure examinations, measurement of body temperature, otoscopy and performance of immunizations did not serve to categorize physicians because all physicians performed them well.[101] As will be described below, in addition to the level at which the standard is set with respect to any given dimension of care, the nature of the dimensions considered in evaluation influences the ability to discriminate levels of care.

Considerations of yield are well illustrated by the adjustments of normative standards to empirical reality in formulating the standards of the AID system of certification of hospital stay. As a rule of thumb, if less than two-thirds of patients are actually discharged by the prescribed day of stay, the standard is considered to be too strict; if 90 to 95 percent of patients are discharged by this day, the standard is too lenient.[23] As the standard becomes more stringent (shorter stay) a greater number of true positives is identified, but only at the expense of including more false positives among the cases under review. Similarly, as the standard becomes less stringent (longer stay), the cases identified are more often true positives but only because many true positives have been missed. The situation is one made familiar by the studies of "sensitivity" and "specificity" in screening tests.[126] It would be interesting to apply the principles and techniques of these studies to the evaluation of some standards of the quality of care.

Explicitness. We have already emphasized that there can be no evaluation without standards. However, standards may be explicit or implicit. This distinction has been considered to be sufficiently important to serve as a basis for classifying case reviews into two categories: those in which the evaluating physician uses internalized standards of what he considers to be good practice, and those in which explicit standards are formulated as a basis or a guide for evaluation.

As we have already pointed out, this two-category classification may obscure a very wide continuum. The studies of Morehead are at one extreme, emphasizing implicit, nondirective criteria. In the study of care received by Teamster families, the assessing physician was simply instructed as follows: "You will use as a yardstick in relation to the quality of care rendered whether you would have treated this particular patient in this particular fashion during this specific hospital admission."[39] At the other extreme are the studies of Peterson and Barsamian [125, 127] and of Richardson [128] wherein a virtually watertight "logic system" is constructed that specifies all the decision rules governing diagnosis and treatment. Given the basic data and the decision rules, assessment can be carried out by computer. Most studies, including the early work of Lembcke,[41-43] fall somewhere in between with respect to degree of specification of explicit criteria. Another intermediate approach is to specify not the precise criteria of what is good or bad practice, but the dimensions of care to be considered and the procedures for evaluation. This approach was used, in part, by Peterson et al.[11] and by Rosenfeld.[100] It is also the basis of the "guides" prepared by the Hospital Utilization Project for use in case review of selected diagnoses as one step in the utilization review sequence (see pages 45 to 50 of Reference 31 for samples of these guides).

Lembcke has proposed certain principles that he believed were generally applicable to the development of criteria regardless of the type of case (Reference 41, pages 648–649):

1. Objectivity—Criteria should be stated in writing with sufficient precision and detail to make them relatively immune to varying interpretations by different individuals.
2. Verifiability—Criteria should be so framed that points on which they rest can be verified by laboratory examination, consultation or documentation.
3. Uniformity—In view of the essential uniformity of the human body and its diseases, criteria should be independent of such factors as size or location of hospital, qualifications of the physician, or social and economic status of patient.
4. Specificity—Criteria should be specific for each kind of disease or operation to be evaluated, and all significant and closely related diseases or operations in the same patient should be considered as a unit.
5. Pertinence—To the greatest extent possible, criteria should be pertinent to the ultimate aim of the medical care being evaluated, and they should be based on results rather than intentions. . . .
6. Acceptability—Criteria should conform with generally accepted standards of good quality as set forth in leading textbooks and articles based on scientific study.

Highly precise and directive standards are associated with the selection of particular diagnostic categories for assessment. But when a representative sample of all the care provided is to be evaluated, little more than general guides can be given to the assessor. Lembcke, who has stressed the need for specific criteria, has had to develop a correspondingly detailed diagnostic classification of pelvic surgery, for example.[41] In addition to diagnostic specificity, explicit standards are associated with the preselection of specific dimensions of care for evaluation. Certain diagnoses, such as short-term, uncomplicated illnesses and surgical operations, lend themselves more readily to this approach. This is evident in Lembcke's attempt to extend his system of audits to nonsurgical diagnoses.[43] The data abstracted under each diagnostic rubric are like descriptions of patterns of management.

EXPLICITNESS

Since there are insufficient normative criteria for decisive evaluation, the alternative used is comparison with a criterion institution.

Payne has been more successful in assembling "criteria" formulated by 15 expert panels concerning approximately 50 diagnoses, medical as well as surgical. For each condition there are a moderate number of criteria which serve as guides for decisions concerning the appropriateness of most or all of the following: indications for admission, indications for office treatment, history required, physical examination, services required (laboratory, roentgenology, special services and therapy), services consistent with diagnosis (laboratory, roentgenology, special services, and therapy), probable length of stay, complications that may extend length of stay, and indications for discharge. The following abstract, giving a number of criteria much reduced from the original, is presented to give the reader a more concrete notion of what is involved in the formulation of standards using this approach (Reference 47, pages 64–65):

Criteria for Urinary Tract Infection

Indications for Admission
    Presence of sepsis (fever, sweat, prostration, chills)
Indications for Office Treatment
    The patient who is uncomfortable but not septic and can pass urine should be treated as an outpatient.
History Required
    Specific reference to . . . frequency of urination . . . obstructive symptoms . . . hematuria . . . incontinence . . . previous urologic disease
Physical Examination
    Specific reference to digital rectal and/or pelvic examination
Services Required for Acutely Ill Patient
    Laboratory
        Urinalysis with stain sediment
    Roentgenology
        Chest roentgenogram
    Special examination
        None
    Therapy
        Institution of antibacterial therapy as soon as possible
Services Consistent with Diagnosis
    Laboratory
        Appropriate tests of renal function
    Roentgenology
        Cystogram
    Special examination
        Cystoscopy
Services Required for Resistant or Recurrent Infection
    History
        As in acute infection
    Physical examination
        Determination of residual urine

Laboratory
> Tuberculin skin test and/or urine culture for tubercle bacilli

Roentgenology
> Intravenous pyelogram and/or retrograde pyelogram

Special examination
> Cystoscopy

Probable Length of Stay
> Diagnostic admission: 72 hours in adults, 5 days in children
> Therapeutic admission: as determined by discharge criteria

Complications That May Extend Length of Stay
> Fistula, neoplasm, congenital anomaly, obstruction, resistant infection, operation, adverse drug reaction.

Indications for Discharge
> Resolution of sepsis
> No correctible factors contributing to infection are present.

Even when the entire set of criteria for urinary tract infection to be found in the original list is considered, it is clear that there is no attempt to cover every possible phase of management. Rather the emphasis falls on key elements of technical management that can usually be readily identified as present or absent by review of the record. Moreover, while the need for reviewer judgment is greatly reduced, it is not entirely removed. For example, the assessor must still judge whether the tests of renal function performed under the heading of Services Consistent with Diagnosis are "appropriate," or whether "no correctible factors contributing to infection are present" at the time of discharge.

Certain consequences derive from the extent to which standards are made explicit and binding upon the assessor. Obviously, the more general and nondirective the standards are, the more one must depend on the interpretations and norms of the person entrusted with the actual assessment of care. With greater specificity, the researcher, the hospital administrator or the medical staff collectively are able to exercise much greater control over the delineation of acceptable standards and the decision to emphasize certain dimensions of care. This allows the introduction of external standards into a situation where the prevalent norms need upgrading and also makes possible the active participation of the hospital staff in the initial development of criteria or in the adaptation of criteria already formulated by external panels of experts to local conditions. Staff participation in the formulation of criteria is considered to be a vitally important feature of the "criteria approach" advocated by Payne. It ensures acceptability of the criteria and of the whole system of quality supervision. It also has an important educational effect. Knowledge of the criteria by the persons who are expected to abide by them is considered to be an important instrument of education, communication and change in behavior.[44]

EXPLICITNESS

Once specific criteria are developed, abstracts or worksheets can be prepared for the physician, usually by the medical record librarian. Payne gives examples of such "worksheets."[46, 47] Prior abstracting should greatly simplify and expedite the process of evaluation. In addition, as Lembcke has claimed, the formulation of highly specific criteria may permit persons with less expertise to evaluate care:

> It is said that with a cookbook, anyone who can read can cook. The same is true, and to about the same extent, of the medical audit using objective criteria; anyone who knows enough medical terminology to understand the definitions and the criteria can prepare the case abstracts and tables for the medical audit. However, the final acceptance, interpretation and application of the findings must be the responsibility of a physician or group of physicians.[42]

With still greater specification of criteria, the entire task can be turned over to a computer.[125, 127, 128]

The specification of standards, though reducing the area within which the judgments of the individual assessor come into play, may be expected to have an important influence on the validity and reliability of judgments concerning the quality of care. Rosenfeld asserts that there is enough experience to indicate that reliability is improved through the introduction of standards (Reference 6, page 48). On the other hand, Morehead *et al.* have raised the important question of whether the reliability obtained through detailed specification of standards may not be gained at the cost of reduced validity:

> Frequently, such criteria force into a rigid framework similar actions or factors which may not be appropriate in a given situation due to the infinite variations in the reaction of the human body to illness.... The study group rejects the assumption that such criteria are necessary to evaluate the quality of medical care. It is their unanimous opinion that it is as important for the surveyors to have flexibility in the judgment of an individual case as it is for a competent physician when confronting a clinical problem in a given patient.[39]

Unfortunately, these various opinions cannot be tested by the results of controlled studies. Peterson *et al.*[11] and Rosenfeld[100] asked the same judges to assess care with and without the use of a structured approach involving some specification of criteria and of scoring methods. The introduction of the more structured and systematic approach appeared to make little difference in the ratings. Indeed, the "qualitative" and "quantitative" ratings in the study by Peterson *et al.* were so similar that they could be used interchangeably. Unreported data by Morehead *et al.*[39] could be analyzed in the same way as those of Rosenfeld[100] to give useful information about the relationship between degree of reliability and method of assessment. The partial data already published suggest that the postreview reliability achieved by Morehead *et al.*, using the most nondirective of approaches, is quite comparable with that obtained by Rosenfeld, who used a more direct technique. On the other hand, Riedel has commented on the higher reliability achieved by the application, in Nassau County hospitals, of Payne's "criteria approach" when contrasted with the "peer judgment" method used by Richardson and his coworkers in Rochester, New York (Reference 25, page 25). The truth of the matter may be that highly skilled, experienced and motivated judges can readily analyze and assess complex clinical situations without the use of explicit criteria. However, explicit standards may be useful for the assessment of less complex clinical situations and by less expert, experienced or motivated judges. Further research to elucidate the merits and limitations of the two approaches is necessary.

Content. In the introductory section to this volume we discussed the definition of quality and presented a view of the many dimensions contained within that definition. For purposes of assessment, general definitions of quality must be further specified and rendered operational. The dimensions of care selected for assessment and the value judgments attached to them constitute an operationalized definition of quality in a given study or system of quality appraisal. It becomes important, therefore, to identify what dimensions are included in an evaluational system and to judge whether they cover the range of dimensions believed necessary to obtain a well-rounded view of quality.

Studies of quality differ with respect to the number of dimensions used and the exhaustiveness with which each dimension is explored. Studies that use many dimensions of care (these may be referred to as "polydimensional") include those of Peterson *et al.*,[11] Rosenfeld,[100] Payne [47] and Lembcke.[41] Morehead gives a brief listing of the dimensions evaluated in the HIP studies of the quality of ambulatory care. These are:

  I. Records
     A. History
     B. Physical examination
     C. Progress notes
     D. Organization of the medical record
     E. Justification of the recorded tentative diagnosis
 II. Diagnostic Management
     A. Time involved in obtaining procedures
     B. Indicated laboratory studies, with minimum of hemoglobin, urinalysis, and serology required in every case
     C. X-ray examinations, with a minimum of chest film required in every case
     D. Indicated consultations
     E. Summary of overall diagnostic handling

CONTENT

   III. Treatment and Follow-up
      A. Therapy
      B. Follow-up laboratory and X-ray studies
      C. Adequacy of follow-up visits
      D. Overall management [40]

In marked contrast are studies in which two or three items are chosen to represent the complex concept of quality. An excellent example of what might be called the "oligodimensional" approach to evaluation is the study by Huntley et al. who evaluated outpatient care using two criteria only: the percent of work-ups that did not include certain routine procedures, and the percent of abnormalities found that were not followed up.[129] To illustrate the fact that classification into "polydimensional" and "oligodimensional" studies does not account for all variants, one might point to the studies of Peterson and Barsamian.[125, 127] These studies concentrate on two basic dimensions—justification of diagnosis and of therapy—but they require complete proof of justification.

We have already pointed out that definitions of quality tend to an excessive preoccupation with traditionally defined dimensions of technical management. Because aspects of preventive, rehabilitative, social and psychological management are generally not represented in the evaluative frame of reference, they do not appear in the standards and criteria formulated. Examples are the intentional exclusion of psychiatric care from the Peterson study [11] and the planned exclusion by the Health Insurance Plan of Greater New York of the patient-physician relationship and of physicians' attitudes from studies of the quality of care.[40] Rosenfeld made a special point of including the performance of specified screening measures among the criteria of superior care; but care was nevertheless labeled "good" without these measures.[100] In the absence of specific instructions to the judges, the study by Morehead et al. includes histories of cases, considered to have received optimal care, in which failure of preventive management could have resulted in serious consequences to the patient.[39]

It would seem self-evident that judgments of quality are incomplete when only a few dimensions are used and decisions about each dimension are made on the basis of partial evidence. But how incomplete they are depends on the extent of homogeneity within the practice of each physician or institution. If practice of all aspects of care is relatively homogeneous, information on relatively few aspects of care may be sufficient to give a reasonably good picture of the quality of care across the board. The phenomena of heterogeneity and homogeneity have been discussed, and the empirical evidence concerning them has been presented, in previous sections of this volume.

One particular aspect, which has not been discussed before, is the relationship of the number and nature of dimensions represented in the standards to the ability of the standards to discriminate among levels of care. Morehead describes the problem in the HIP evaluations as follows:

> The methods described were recognized to be a crude index at best. They served their purpose well in delineating those physicians providing medical care of an unacceptable level of quality, but were not so efficient in separating the *average* from the *good* or *excellent* performances. For example, a physician who had given a patient with a peptic ulcer an adequate basic work-up, repeat hemoglobin levels, and X-rays when indicated would have received a score of 100. But another physician, who, in addition to all the services mentioned, had arranged for the patient to discuss his diet with the consultant-nutritionist, had involved the social worker in possible problems existing in the patient's home, or had referred the patient to a psychiatrist if indicated, would have received the same score.[40]

This observation suggests that there might be a hierarchical order in physician performance and points to the need for further research into the nature of physician performance with respect to the many dimensions of care.

Measurement Scales

The construction of a scale that indicates the position of a physician or institution on a continuum from best to worst is often a necessary tool in research on the quality of care. One may wish to explore the relationships between structure and the quality of care, or between the quality of care and outcome; and, for these purposes, a single quantitative measure of quality would be a convenient measure of change in one of the three basic variables.

In administratively oriented systems of quality review, the whole problem of scaling may be circumvented because the object, most often, is not to arrive at a measure of quality, but to identify normatively aberrant elements of performance and to correct them. Attaching a label which represents the quality of management of a case or the overall performance of a provider may, therefore, be irrelevant and unnecessary. But certain administrative studies may require the construction of measurement scales, and the administrator would do well to have some understanding of the problems involved.

All scales that purport to measure the quality of care are ordinal in nature. In other words, they arrange examples of care in an order from best to worst; but the intervals between one position on the scale and the next are not equal. The difference between "fair" and "poor" is not the same as that between "fair" and "good"; nor can one say that a physician who scores 80 points is twice as good as one who scores 40. The inequality of intervals is a characteristic of ordinal scales in general, and must be kept in mind in all studies of quality.

The ability to discriminate different levels of performance depends, in part, on the number of intervals in the scale. The examples cited in the paragraph above illustrate the two basic variants in scale construction. Some studies of quality use a small number of divisions to classify care into categories such as "excellent," "good," "fair" or "poor." A provider's relative position in a set can then be further specified by computing the percent of cases in each scale category. Other studies assign scores to performance of specified components of care and cumulate these to obtain a numerical index usually ranging from 0–100. These two methods of scaling correspond to the categories of "ranking" and "scoring" described by Sheps as follows:

> In general, qualitative judgments are expressed through either ranking or scoring. In ranking, a number of units are placed by each judge in order of this preference and the various ranks analyzed for consistency. In scoring, a scale of quality is established and each judge assigns the score that he considers appropriate. These techniques may be combined in various ways. Thus, individual scores can be given on quality in different clinical fields, and findings combined into one overall score. The subjects may then be ranked according to the scores obtained.[9]

The use of a simple scale with a few divisions is defended on several grounds. It is claimed, by those who prefer it, that any greater degree of precision is not possible with present methods. Some have even reduced the categories to two: optimal and less than optimal.[38,39] Clute has used three, of which the middle one was acknowledged to be doubtful or indeterminate.[101] The simple scale also appears to deal more realistically with the all-or-none aspect of medical care. Care can be good in many of its parts, and disastrously inadequate in the aggregate—due to a vital error in one component. This means that simple addition of subscores to obtain a total score may not be a valid procedure in some instances.

The major disadvantage of the use of a scale with few divisions is the possible loss of information and a lower ability to discriminate.[125] This, in turn, depends on whether the number of divisions is smaller than the precision in assessment would make possible. We have run full circle to the first argument in favor of scales with few divisions.

Those who use numerical subscores, which are cumulated to a total score, obviously believe it is in this way possible to preserve valid information that the few-interval scales appear to throw away. The subscores, presented in detail, also give information on performance with respect to aspects or dimensions of care which constitute the whole. In Morehead's view, "Weighting and scoring have advantages when large numbers of cases are involved, and the study objectives envision establishing priorities for administrative action. It allows for ready assessment of areas in need of corrective action—weakness on the part of specific groups of physicians [and in] areas such as follow-up, records, minimal use of laboratory data, etc."[40a] She does not make clear precisely why this is so. Perhaps part of the advantage comes from the impression of precision and objectivity that is conveyed by numerical scores (Mindel Sheps in Reference 6, page 22).

The construction of numerical scores raises certain problems of measurement that are implicit in all scales, including those with few intervals. One of these is the question of whether the subscores can be simply added, or whether some type of weighting must be done; and if other than equal weights are to be used, on what basis the weights are to be determined. These considerations are of a general nature and apply whenever subparts are to be combined. They are relevant to the summation of various aspects of care. They also apply to the combination of various diagnostic categories such as major and minor surgery, or surgery of different grades of difficulty within the "major" category.

At present, weighting is handled in an arbitrary or intuitive manner. Peterson et al.,[11] for example, arrive at the following scale: clinical history 30, physical examination 34, use of laboratory aids 26, therapy 9, preventive medicine 6, clinical records 2, total 107. In the HIP studies [40] the following weights were used: records 30, diagnostic work-up 40, treatment and follow-up 30, total 100. Peterson et al. say: "Greatest importance is attached to the process of arriving at a diagnosis since, without a diagnosis, therapy cannot be rational. Furthermore, therapy is in the process of constant change, while the form of history and physical examination has changed very little over the years." [11] Equally persuasive arguments could probably be made on behalf of the weights adopted in the HIP studies of ambulatory care. However, Morehead recognizes the problem as follows:

> The arbitrary assignment of weights to different components of care was one of the most difficult areas to defend against criticism of the group physicians. In large part it was dictated by the volume of material to be studied; e.g. 4,070 cases for the family physicians alone. . . . Administratively, the weighting system was invaluable; but it continued to present problems, not all of which were ever resolved.[40]

Another problem that is highlighted by the attempt to construct numerical scores is the lack of independence among the elements of practice to which subscores are attached. For example, sufficiency of treatment depends on the adequacy of the preceding diagnosis.[40] This means that diagnosis and treatment cannot be scored independently. The inability of the usual numerical scores to deal with the all-or-none property of medical care, to which we have already referred, is an extension of the problem of lack of independence among subparts. Finally, one might refer again to the difficulties that were encountered in conveying the meaning of numerical scores to physicians in the HIP studies of quality.[40]

A variety of solutions, or approaches to possible solutions, have been proposed to help handle some of the problems of scaling mentioned above. In attempting to deal with the choice of arbitrary or intuitive weights, Peterson *et al.* sought empirical verification through the use of factor analysis:

> If the factor analysis method were accepted as final judgment, however, the results indicate that case history should have had slightly more influence in the final index, laboratory considerably less, and preventive medicine and records somewhat more. On the other hand, when indexes of overall capacity for goodness were constructed using the factorial weights, the resultant values were practically identical, correlationwise, with the judgment type of quantitative index employed in the analysis. Consequently, the indexes by factorial methods were used only as confirmatory evidence that the quantitative index appeared to be satisfactory. (Reference 11, footnote, pages 14 and 15.)

Mindel Sheps has suggested that, rather than starting out with *a priori* weights, a statistical technique called discriminant analysis [130] might be used to derive the appropriate weights from the data themselves (Reference 6, page 23).

The problem of weights is related to the more general problem of value of items of information or procedures in the medical care process. Rimoldi *et al.* used the frequency with which specified items of information were employed in the solution of a test problem as a measure of that item's value.[131] Williamson had experts classify designated procedures, in a specified diagnostic test setting, on a scale ranging from "very helpful" to "very harmful." Individual performance in the test was then rated using quantitative indices of "efficiency," "proficiency" and overall "competence," depending on the frequency and nature of the procedures used.[132]

Perhaps the simplest solution to the problem of weighting is not to attempt to combine the subparts at all, but to score each part separately. For example, there could be a separate score for each of major and minor surgery, and even for subgroups within the category of major surgery. This is especially appropriate when the data are for administrative use and the object, for example, is to determine the assignment of surgical privileges (Mindel Sheps in Reference 6, page 20).

The problem of interdependence of subparts is more difficult to circumvent unless it is demonstrated that there is considerable homogeneity in provider performance with respect to all the subparts. If this were so, the problem would not arise. Unfortunately there appears to be enough variability, at least in individual examples of care, to keep the issue very much alive.

Morehead describes as follows the problem of interdependence:

> Consideration was given to the development of interlocking scores; i.e., if the diagnostic area failed to rate x number of points, then the therapy area could not exceed x number of points. It was felt, however, that this would be an additional artifact to explain to the clinician. To a certain extent the 20 points allocated for a summary of diagnostic handling were used to serve this purpose.[40]

Mindel Sheps seems to be advocating a similar approach when she describes a system, likened to the branching of a tree, in which the score for each step in the process of care is dependent on the score given to the step that is its necessary precursor (Reference 6, pages 21–22).

Rosenfeld has attempted to meet the problem of loss of information in nonnumerical scales, as well as allowing for the all-or-none property of care, by using a system of assigning qualitative scores to component parts of care and an overall qualitative score based on arbitrary rules for combining the subparts.[100]

In the HIP study of ambulatory care, special attempts were made to assure appropriate interpretation of the quantitative scores to the participating medical groups. The quantitative scores were arbitrarily translated into descriptive equivalents as follows: 45 or less poor, 46–60 below average, 61 or higher acceptable. Perhaps the most useful feature, in terms of communicating with physicians, was the inclusion of a narrative justification given by the surveyor for his rating in each case.[40]

Reliability, Validity and Bias

Reliability, validity and bias are major considerations in studies of quality, where so much depends on judgment even when explicit and directive standards are used.

Reliability refers to the ability of two observers, or more, to examine the same data and arrive at the same judgment concerning the quality of care. It also includes the ability of any person to examine one set of data two or more times and arrive at identical judgments. The reliability of a method of assessment, then, is the degree to which results are reproducible when the assessment is repeated by one person or different persons.

Bias refers to a consistent tendency for one assessor to judge care to be better or worse than does another assessor who examines the same data. It also includes other systematic tendencies that affect the ratings but are unrelated to the merits of the cases themselves. Examples are: rating cases that are reviewed earlier lower than those that are reviewed later, or rating care rendered by certain providers, or categories of providers, lower than those rendered by others. There is always variability in measurement, but this is expected to be random and, therefore, to even out in the long run. Bias exists only if there is a consistent leaning in one direction or another.

Validity refers to whether a test measures what it purports to measure. Does the review of certain elements of performance, for example, actually measure quality? If two providers are assigned different ratings, do they, in fact, provide care at different levels of quality?

Determination of the degree of reliability, validity and bias is an essential element in the development of any instrument for measurement or evaluation. The definitions provided above, which are not intended to be rigorous, indicate the manner in which these characteristics are measured. Reliability is measured by comparing the results of repeated examinations of the same data by the same person or by different persons. "The reliability of qualitative judgments can be tested and subjected to statistical analysis."[9] Bias is tested through setting up special comparisons, the nature of which depends on the type of bias that one suspects. For example, if one imagines that the assessor tends to favor cases coming from a given hospital, the ratings may be compared on two similar batches of case records, one with, and one without, obscuring the identity of the hospital.

Validity is generally much more difficult to establish. When a method of assessment is shown to be reliable and free from bias, it is often presumed to be valid because measurement cannot be valid unless it is also reliable and unbiased. Unfortunately, a method of assessment can be reliable and free of bias and yet not valid, because while the method of assessment might be good, it may nevertheless measure something different from what was intended. The validity of a new method of measurement is usually tested against an existing measure accepted or known to have superior validity. In the assessment of medical care, all methods of measurement ultimately derive their validity from the extent to which the ratings they assign to instances of care are related to the end results of that care as represented in health and well-being. The reader is referred to previous sections of this volume for discussions of the validating function of end results and of the variability in validity of the standards used in assessment of the process of care.*

The literature on the assessment of quality identifies a number of factors that influence primarily the reliability and, secondarily, the validity of assessment. These include the accuracy and veracity of the basic data on which assessment rests, the degree of specification in the standards for assessment, the qualifications of judges used in case review and the use of many judges to review each case. Some of these factors have been discussed in previous sections to which the reader is referred. In the section on Sources of Information, the reader will find a discussion of the accuracy of claim forms and record abstracts, as well as of the completeness and veracity of information in the record itself. In the section on Standards, there is a discussion of the effects which the explicit formulation of standards is thought to have on reliability and validity. A summary of the empirical findings is also reported. Still to be examined are the considerations relevant to the qualifications of judges, their number and the manner of their use.

In considering the qualifications of judges, the administrator must remind himself once again what the purpose and methods of evaluation are to be. In the administrative setting, where one of the major functions is the educational effect of the assessment of quality on the assessor as well as on the person subject to assessment, and when the method selected is the internal audit of medical records, the choice might well be to allow for rotation of the hospital staff on the medical audit committee. On the other hand, when an external audit of cases is to be done to determine what, if anything, is wrong with the care provided in any organization, the competence, experience, impartiality and prestige of the evaluator become matters of central concern. As we have already described, these qualities are likely to be called upon to a greater extent if no explicit standards have been formulated and the assessor must rely on his own standards and clinical acumen. The choice of assessor is even more critical when the evaluation of care is part of a carefully planned research study that requires high levels of precision in measurement. There are, in addition, matters of work habits, motivation and aptitude which often become apparent only after there has been some experience with the work of the assessor. These issues are well summarized by Morehead:

> Outstanding clinicians with no prior association with the Plan were selected for each of the fields to be studied. All of the team members were affiliated with teaching institutions and, to avoid the problem of ivory tower standards, were also engaged in clinical practice.... It is obvious that the status of the reviewer as seen by his professional colleagues is very important. Younger

---

* This discussion of reliability, validity and bias is neither rigorous nor complete. Elinson deals lucidly with this and other aspects of measurement in a brief chapter to which reference has been made in another context.[97] The interested reader may also turn to the chapters in Kerlinger's text on Behavioral Research.[188]

physicians would have been more readily available, in relation to both time and money; but it was felt that regardless of how competent they might be, their findings would be subject to question where ratings of unsatisfactory were given. This is not to say that all senior physicians with outstanding reputations make good surveyors. One outstanding New York clinician and teacher, instead of basing his evaluations on how he would have handled a particular case himself, would invariably address himself first to "Was the patient helped by his hospital stay?" . . . and then to the even less desirable: "Was this patient harmed by his hospital stay?" Problems were also encountered with the type of physician who found the tradition of not criticizing professional colleagues so strong that he was unable to give an unfavorable rating even when his summaries contained references to inappropriate and ill-advised procedures identical to those made by surveyors who gave unsatisfactory ratings. Surveyors with highly specialized interests that interfered with an overall view of the patient's problems were also occasionally encountered; they concentrated on the aspect of the disease that was of interest to them and tended to ignore important concomitant events. The surveyors who were considered most suitable for this activity were generally senior clinicians, with a teaching appointment in one of the City's medical schools, and were also engaged in clinical practice. The majority had extensive experience with the review of clinical records either in a supervisory capacity in their hospital activities or as surveyors for the Joint Commission on Accreditation, or both (Reference 40, pages 3 and 17–18).

As we have already discussed, there is reason to believe that the reliability and validity of judgments may be increased by the prior formulation of guidelines and criteria, provided they are not rigidly applied. Furthermore, it may be useful to train the assessors through the evaluation of a set of test cases with subsequent discussion of the reasons for downgrading the record. This assures the researcher that the procedure is well understood and the criteria, if these have been spelled out, are properly and uniformly applied. When two or more assessors are asked to evaluate each record independently, it has been customary to arrange for joint discussions of the several ratings so that some commonality is established.

The precision of measurement is much improved by using independent repetition. The same assessor could repeat his own assessments, if it were possible to be certain that he is not influenced by the results of his previous assessments. Generally, more than one assessor can be used, and the precision attained depends on the number of assessments made on each case.[134] The use of several assessors is likely to reduce bias.[134] It also provides a margin of safety against the occasional breakdown of an assessor, resulting in a totally aberrant group of assessments that might otherwise go undetected.[100]

A final approach to improving reliability and validity is to use group decision in the evaluation of quality. The various hospital review committees obviously function in this way. In the New York Academy of Medicine study of perinatal mortality, the evaluation of each case involved the participation of a number of staff members as well as a subcommittee of 21 persons: nine obstetricians, nine pediatricians and three pathologists.

> The reports prepared by the investigators were examined by the original Director, who selected for review by the Committee on Neonatal Mortality those which were not clear cut. These were referred to panels constituted from the Subcommittee. There were several such panels, each consisting of one obstetrician, one pediatrician, and one pathologist. The panels reviewed all the referred cases for preventability, the factors of responsibility, and the causes of death. The investigators were present at the meetings of these panels to supply additional information from their notes. The ultimate results represent the composite judgment of the groups after differences of opinion had been resolved through a full discussion (Reference 84, page 4).

In the second study of hospital care received by Teamster families, Morehead used two assessors to rate each case independently. The assessors then met to discuss all cases and, in almost all instances, arrived at a single joint rating for the case. Although the "committee" approach appears to be eminently reasonable, and in keeping with democratic tradition, its value in handling the problem of reliability does not seem to have been the subject of much study. This is in contrast to the use of independent replication, which is supported by a considerable body of statistical methods. Sheps comments as follows on the distinction between the two methods:

> As already emphasized, the use of these techniques depends on replication, that is, on securing at least two separate evaluations of the same set of units. This is not the same as asking a committee to make a combined appraisal. Only through separate evaluations is it possible to assess the consistency of the individual judgments and to arrive at a relatively unbiased estimate. The value assigned results from combining the different judgments, and is more reliable and objective than the opinion of a single individual. A committee of experts would emerge with one final appraisal, but this would not allow the internal checking suggested. It is even possible with such a panel that one or two members could influence the others so that the final assessment would not be truly a consensus.[9]

Reliability—It would be useful to review some of the empirical studies that have attempted to establish the reliability level of currently available methods for appraising quality of care and appropriateness of length of stay. Those studies that deal particularly with the possible effect of specification of standards have already been described. In addition, several studies dealing with the extent of agreement among judges give the impression that it is considered to be at an acceptable level. Peterson *et al.*, on the basis of 14 observer revisits, judged agreement to be high enough for all the observations to be pooled together after adjustment for observer bias in one of the six major divisions of care.[11] In the study by Daily and Morehead,

RELIABILITY

"several cross-checks were made between the two interviewing internists by having them interview the same physicians. The differences in the scores of the family physicians based on these separate ratings did not exceed seven percent."[37] Rosenfeld paid considerable attention to testing reliability, and devised mathematical indices of "agreement" and "dispersion" to measure it. These indicate a fair amount of agreement, but a precise evaluation is difficult since no other investigator is known to have used these same measures.[100] Morehead et al., in the second study of medical care received by Teamster families, report initial agreement between two judges in assigning care to one of two classes in 78 percent of cases. This was raised to 92 percent following reevaluation of disagreements by the two judges.[39]

As mentioned in a previous section, the reliability of judgments based on record abstracts was tested in the study of the office practice of New York internists. Ten physicians reviewed independently the same 21 abstracts:

> The only instruction given these ten physicians was to review the abstract, and on the basis of what what was recorded, to grade the quality of care . . . (on a scale from 1 "excellent" to 4 "very poor"). No guidance as to specifics for evaluating the quality was given. The grading was a result of the individual subjective evaluations of ten physicians with widely different backgrounds. . . . Despite the absence of specific grading criteria, there was good agreement among the group. Over half the judges were in perfect agreement on the grade given 13 of the 21 abstracts. When the number of judges who marked an abstract 1 or 2 (good) was compared with the number who marked it 3 or 4 (not good), it was found that in three cases all judges were unanimous, in three cases all but one judge agreed, and in 20 of the 21 cases a clear majority of the judges agreed. There was only one case where the judges were equally divided.[104]

By contrast to between-judge reliability, very little has been reported about the reliability of repeated judgments of quality made by the same person. To test within-observer variation, Peterson et al. asked two observers to revisit four of their own previously visited physicians. The level of agreement was lower within observers than between observers, partly because revisits lasted a shorter period of time and related, therefore, to a smaller sample of practice.[11]

The reasons for disagreement among judges throw some light on the problems of evaluation and the prospects of achieving greater reliability. Rosenfeld found that "almost half the differences were attributable to situations not covered adequately by standards, or in which the standards were ambiguous. In another quarter differences developed around questions of fact, because one consultant missed a significant item of information in the record. It would therefore appear that with revised standards, and improved methods of orienting consultants, a substantially higher degree of agreement could be achieved."[100] Less than a quarter of the disagreements contained differences of opinion with regard to the requirements of management.

Given the many unsettled issues in medicine, differences of opinion are inevitable. Morehead *et al.* reported that in about half the cases of initial disagreement "there was agreement on the most serious aspect of the patient's care, but one surveyor later agreed that he had not taken into account corollary aspects of patient care."[39] Difficulty in adhering to the rating categories, or failure to note all the facts, were the basis of other disagreements. Of the small number of unresolved disagreements (eight percent of all admissions and 36 percent of initial disagreements) more than half were due to honest differences of opinion regarding the clinical handling of the problem. The remainder arose out of interpreting inadequate records, or from the technical problems of where to assess unsatisfactory care in a series of admissions.[39]

There have been several studies of the reliability of judgments concerning the need for admission to the hospital and justification of length of stay. The second study of hospital care received by Teamster families included tests of the reliability of judgments concerning the need for admission to the hospital in each case.[39] Browning has reported a study based on the independent review, by two physicians, of 1763 discharge records in the seven general hospitals of Rochester, New York.[135] Each assessor answered five questions with respect to each case:

1. Was the patient admitted for diagnostic studies not requiring hospitalization?
2. Could the patient's hospital stay have been shortened by earlier discharge or transfer to another facility?
3. Was the hospital stay prolonged by unnecessary delay between admission and surgery?
4. Was the hospital stay prolonged by unnecessary delay in consultation?
5. Was the hospital stay prolonged by unnecessary delay in ordering or receiving lab studies, X-rays or some other service?

The answers to these questions will be given below.

The interest created by the Browning study in Rochester led to another study by Zimmer, based in the University of Rochester Hospital and characterized by some interesting refinements of study design.[136] Four physicians were asked to review the record of each patient while still in hospital, and to judge whether hospital stay was or was not required. Two of the four judges were restricted to information in the patient's record, whereas the other two were permitted to interview the patient's physician and to examine the patient if they felt these procedures were necessary to arrive at a decision.

RELIABILITY

For the reader's convenience, the major findings of the three studies referred to above have been assembled in Table 1. The key points are summarized in Table 2:

Table 1. Reliability of Judgments Concerning the Appropriateness of Hospital Use in Specified Studies.

Source of Data and Nature of Study	Judgments	Numbers	Percent of Total Cases	Percent of Questionable Cases
Morehead (39): Necessity for admission. 2 judges.	2 yes, 0 no *	212	74	..
	1 yes, 1 no	36	12	47
	0 yes, 2 no	40	14	53
Browning (135): Various aspects in improper use of hospital services. 2 judges.	2 yes, 0 no	1442	82	..
	1 yes, 1 no	256	15	80
	0 yes, 2 no	65	14	20
Zimmer (136): Need for continued stay based on chart review. 2 judges.	2 yes, 0 no	289	81	..
	1 yes, 1 no	53	15	76
	0 yes, 2 no	16	4	23
Zimmer (136): Need for continued stay based on chart review with opportunity to interview physician and examine patient. 2 judges.	2 yes, 0 no	305	85	..
	1 yes, 1 no	38	11	72
	0 yes, 2 no	15	5	28
Zimmer (136): Need for continued stay based on all observations combined. 4 judges.	4 yes, 0 no	263	73	..
	3 yes, 1 no	59	16	62
	2 yes, 2 no	20	6	21
	1 yes, 3 no	10	3	11
	0 yes, 4 no	6	2	6

* "Yes" means hospital use is justified and "no" that it is not justified.

The findings of these studies indicate that some question was raised, by one or more judges, concerning the appropriateness of hospital use in 15 to 27 percent of cases. The findings on agreement depend on which of two measures of agreement one wishes to consider. If one includes full agreement on appropriate as well as inappropriate use, as a percent of all cases (column 2 of Table 2), the picture is

Table 2. Summary of Reliability of Judgments in Specified Studies.

Source and Nature of Study	Percent of Cases Questioned by One or More Judges*	All Full Agreement as Percent of All Cases*	Full Agreement on Inappropriate Use as Percent of Questionable Cases*
Morehead (39): Two judges.	26	88	53
Browning (135): Two judges.	18	86	20
Zimmer (136): Charts only. Two judges.	19	85	23
Zimmer (136): Charts with supplementation. Two judges.	15	89	28
Zimmer (136): Pooled data. Four judges.	27	73	6

* The manner in which the percentages are computed is described in the following paragraph of the text.

very good. Agreement between two judges ranges from 85–89 percent of cases, and agreement among four judges is 73 percent. These high values of agreement occur mainly because the percent of cases questioned is rather small. If one allows for this by considering only cases that have been questioned by one or more judges, and computes the proportion of such cases in which there is full agreement that hospital use is inappropriate, the picture is not so encouraging (column 3). Agreement between two judges ranges from 20 to 53 percent, and complete agreement among four judges is only six percent.

A study reported by the Nassau County Medical Society indicates the extent of agreement on appropriateness of admission and length of stay using explicit criteria similar to those developed by Payne.[193] Systematic samples of cases falling in seven diagnostic categories were drawn in each of five participating hospitals. The cases were rated by a utilization committee in each hospital using uniform criteria developed by panels of local physicians. All the cases were later reviewed and rated independently by Dr. Payne at the University of Michigan using the identical criteria. In addition to the use of explicit criteria, this study differs from the others described above by including the comparison of internal versus external judgments. It should also be noted that the cases drawn are not a probability sample of any definable universe. The findings in Tabulation III-2 should be interpreted with these characteristics in mind (Reference 193, Tables 1a, 1b and 2a).

RELIABILITY

Tabulation III-2.

Aspect of Care Evaluated	Percent of Cases Questioned by One or Both Parties	All Full Agreement as Percent of All Cases	Full Agreement on Inappropriate Use as Percent of Questionable Cases
Appropriateness of admission	5% (1208) *	96% (1208)	25% (64)
Length of stay	34% (1207)	72% (1207)	30% (408)

* Bases for the percentages are shown in parentheses. The data for appropriateness of admission include two cases rated "not ascertained" by the hospital utilization committee and which could not be allocated to any of the agreement-disagreement categories constructed from the data in the source reference.

The above findings suggest that there is greater ambiguity in defining and applying normative standards for length of stay than for appropriateness of admission. The relative strictness of internal, as compared with external review will be discussed in a subsequent section of this volume.

The study by Browning includes a subclassification of the nature of inappropriate use as indicated by the answers to the five questions listed on page 87.

Tabulation III-3.

Reason for Inappropriate Use	Percent of Cases Questioned by One or More Judges *	All Full Agreement as Percent of All Cases *	Full Agreement on Inappropriate Use as Percent of Questionable Cases
Diagnostic admission not requiring hospitalization	4	97	22 (74)
Shorten hospital stay by earlier transfer	7	95	27 (123)
Delay between admission and surgery	2	98	31 (42)
Delay in consultation	1	99	5 (19)
Delay in X-ray, lab, etc.	4	97	3 (63)

* The base for percentages in columns 1 and 2 is 1763 cases. The bases for the percentages in column 3 are given in parentheses.

These findings by Browning raise some intriguing questions. Why, for example, is agreement on questionable cases so much lower in the last two categories? Much further work remains to be done to confirm the findings and to elucidate their causes.

Zimmer investigated the effect of certain factors on the extent of agreement among judges. As might be expected, the longer the hospital stay, the more likely there is to be agreement that further stay is inappropriate. The more interesting finding concerns the possible effect on agreement of the opportunity to seek information additional to that in the patient's record. Those pairs of physicians who based their judgments on the records only did not achieve a level of agreement significantly different from the pairs of physicians who were permitted to seek additional information through interviewing the patient's physician or examining the patient. This finding is significant because of the difference of opinion, discussed in a previous section, concerning supplementation of the record by interviews with the managing physician. Unfortunately, the Zimmer findings are not conclusive, partly because the records in a teaching hospital are likely to be unusually complete, and partly because it is not known to what extent the judges who were permitted to do so did, in fact, seek additional information from the patient's physician or through examination of the patient. The conclusion is still: "Not proven."

Validity—In contrast to studies of reliability, direct tests of the validity of methods of quality assessment are very unusual. It was suggested above that the validity of any given method of assessing quality can be tested against a method believed to be of superior validity. This rule, plus the general agreement that exists with respect to any specified outcome, leads one to the reasonable expectation that assessments of process can be validated by concurrent assessment of end results and that evaluations of structure can be validated by evaluation of process or end results. Similarly, within each category (structure, process or outcome), one might expect assessments based on one dimension, or a few, to be validated by comparison with those methods of measurement that are more exhaustive and use many more dimensions of care in the scheme for assessment.

The literature of medical care includes many studies that explore the relationships between elements of structure, process and outcome, in all possible pairs. A thorough familiarity with these studies is essential for the medical care administrator. However, the studies are not designed as tests to validate methods of assessment. One exception is a study by Makover in which he sets out to determine specifically the relationship between multifactorial assessments of structure and of process in the same medical groups associated with

BIAS

the Health Insurance Plan of Greater New York.[36, 137] The 26 groups studied were distributed as shown in Tabulation III-4.

Tabulation III-4.

The Quality of the Groups as Judged by Conformity to Standards	The Quality of the Groups as Judged by Process Characteristics (Review of Records)	
	Low	High
Low	10	3
High	3	10

Makover concludes as follows:

> It was found that the medical groups that achieved higher quality ratings by the method used in this study were those that, in general, adhered more closely to HIP's Minimum Medical Standards [See reference 138]. However, the exceptions were sufficiently marked, both in number and degree, to induce one to question the reliability of one or the other rating methods when applied to any one medical group. It would seem that further comparison of these two methods of rating is clearly indicated.[36]

Bias—Several studies of the quality of medical care contain empirical information on the nature and extent of bias. Peterson *et al.* discovered that one of their two observers generally awarded higher ratings in the assessment of performance of physical examination, but not in the other areas of care that were under scrutiny.[11] Rosenfeld showed that, of two assessors, one regularly awarded lower ratings to the same cases assessed by both.[100] An examination of individual cases of disagreement in the study by Morehead *et al.* reveals that, in the medical category, the same assessor rated the care at a lower level in 11 out of 12 instances of disagreement. For surgical cases, one surveyor rated the care lower than the other in all eight instances of disagreement. The impression gained, from examining the reasons for disagreement on medical cases, is that one of the judges had a special interest in cardiology and was more conservative in the management of such cases.[39]

The clear indication of these findings is that bias must be accepted as the rule rather than the exception, and that studies of quality must be designed with this in mind. In the Rosenfeld study, for example, either of the two raters used for each area of practice would have ranked the several hospitals in the same order, even though one was consistently more generous than the other.[100] The Clute study of general practice in Canada, on the other hand, has been criticized for comparing the quality of care in two geographic areas when different observers examined the care in the two areas in question.[139] Although the author was aware of this problem and devised methods for comparing the performance of the observers in the two geographic areas, the basic weakness remains.

Predetermined order or regularity in the process of study may be associated with bias. Therefore, some carefully planned procedures for randomization may have to be introduced into the research design. The study by Peterson *et al.* appears to be one of the few to have paid attention to this factor.[11] Another source of bias, as we have mentioned, may be the assessor's knowledge of the managing physician's identity or of the hospital in which care was given. The question of removing identifying features from charts under review has been raised, but little is known about the feasibility of this procedure and its effects on the ratings assigned.[106] Still another type of bias may result from parochial standards and criteria of practice that may develop in and around certain institutions or "schools" of medical practice. To the extent that this is true, or suspected to be true, appropriate precautions need to be taken in the recruitment and allocation of judges.

It is necessary to conclude this section by once again reminding the administrator about the need to adjust the nature and precision of assessment to the uses to which it is to be put. It is true that questions of reliability, validity and bias are central to all measurement and are therefore of concern to the administrator. If nothing else, the administrator must understand the limitations of the assessments of quality that are performed under the administrative umbrella. However, it is equally true that for most administrative uses, a reasonable level of accuracy is sufficient. It is believed that currently available methods of assessment qualify as acceptable in these respects. In particular, Morehead comments that although the use of multiple judges is a useful research technique, it is too costly for routine application. "In operating programs, particularly where cost is always a consideration, the use of one surveyor would seem to suffice; the problem of clinical differences of opinion between highly trained physicians in the same field does not affect the overall findings and recommendations."[40] Riedel believes that although multiple reviews are quite costly for routine application, it is relatively inexpensive and desirable to have multiple reviews on a sample basis to monitor the review system. The size of the sample would be dependent on the variability of opinions expressed by the multiple judges.[180a]

Indices of Medical Care

Although there is a prevalent notion that "indices" may be used to evaluate the quality of medical care, there is some lack of clarity concerning what an index is and how its use might differ from other approaches to assessment.

Sheps ranks the use of indices as the second of four approaches to evaluation, describing it as follows:

> The second approach to quality uses indexes intended to reflect one or more elements of performance. Indexes may be defind as "one or a set of measures ... used to measure indirectly the incidence of a characteristic that is not directly measurable." [140] Patient care is such a characteristic. Its quality cannot be measured quantitatively, except by the arbitrary allotment of a certain number of points to a qualitative judgment. It is difficult to define; it is complex and intangible. It is therefore natural that much of the effort to evaluate this quality has been focused on the development of indexes. . . .[9]

A list of examples is given in Sheps' paper.

Myers has listed and criticized some of the traditional indices used in the evaluation of hospital care. These include rates of total and postoperative mortality, complications, postoperative infection, Caesarean section, consultation and removal of normal tissue at operation.[141] One notes, from these examples, that the notion of an "index" is extended beyond the "elements of performance" listed by Sheps and includes intermediate and ultimate end results. Donabedian has extended the concept even further by adding elements of structure to the list of "indicators" which he has assembled.[5]

It becomes clear, then, that an "index" is an item of information pertaining to structure, process or outcome. Very often it belongs under the categories of "procedural end points" or "intermediate outcomes" that we have identified in a previous section. The chief requirement is that it be easily, sometimes routinely, measurable and reasonably reliable and valid.

Nothing that has been said so far differentiates the use of indices from the statistical display and analysis systems that explore and monitor the elements of process and end results which we have described in a previous section of this volume. The fact that elements of structure can also serve as indices of the quality of medical care is simply an extension rather than a differentiating characteristic.[142, 143] The distinguishing characteristic is to be found in the Hagood definition quoted by Sheps: The index measures indirectly what is not measured directly because direct measurement is impossible, or difficult, or costly, or, for some other reason, impractical to do.[140] This means that the measure of any element of structure, process or outcome becomes an index only when it is used inferentially. Each item counted or measured [9] can therefore be used in two ways: as a measure of itself and as an indicator of other phenomena correlated with itself. It is only when used in the second way that it becomes an "index."

For example, when we determine the autopsy rate at a hospital we obtain a *direct* indication of the ability of the hospital to obtain ultimate diagnostic confirmation in fatal illness and of its ability to provide certain educational experiences to physicians and trainees. But when we *infer* from the low autopsy rate that the hospital is not likely to provide good care, we are using this item of information as an index of something other than itself. Whether the inference is valid depends on how well it correlates with other elements of care that collectively constitute the complex notion of quality. That inferential use is what actually defines the concept of "index" is even more clearly demonstrated when an element of structure, for example the physician-client ratio, is considered to mean "good" care.

The validity of the inferential use of certain items of information is largely a matter of definition and can be categorized as "construct validity." [97, 133] But in many cases, validity must rest on empirical demonstration of relationships, preferably of a causal nature.[1] Unfortunately, such empirical confirmation is not easy to find. Morehead provides one of the few examples of empirical testing of indices in the literature on the evaluation of quality:

> During the course of these [Teamsters' Union] studies, extensive efforts were made to develop indices of patient care from the records that might lead to a simplified and more standardized way of obtaining evaluations of patient care. A registered nurse on the study staff, with extensive experience in working with and abstracting medical records, tabulated many items of patient care in equivalent cases. Many attempts were made to correlate such items with the surveyor's rating. The items ranged from patient identification data to salient factors in the history, laboratory and X-ray findings, to confirmation of pathology reports and other characteristics of the hospital stay. This was done for every group of diagnostic cases, from both studies combined, where more than 10 cases of a similar diagnosis were found. The results were not encouraging, as in general the reasons for adverse judgment were unique for the particular patient and were not identified by the indices no matter how detailed they were. This also had been the experience of the first audit, where the surveyor of cases of diabetes mellitus had, in addition to the form where he summarized his opinion and judgments, an extensive check-list with specific items relating to this disease up to and including strength and scheduling of medications. No profitable use, however, was ever made of these data despite repeated attempts to do so. The only suggestive relationship that occurred was in cases of peptic ulcer surgery, where those with less than favorable ratings all had ulcer history of less than one year, in contrast to those of longer duration whose ratings were more satisfactory. Even here, however, the short duration of the history was not always the major cause for the lower ratings.[40]

The Morehead verdict on the usefulness of indices, while it deserves serious attention, cannot, of course, be taken as final. We have already indicated in the discussion of statistical display and analysis, and in subsequent sections, the manner in which items of information on elements of performance and on end results can be used to monitor the occurrence of changes in the care-providing system, and to screen out cases that require further scrutiny. The use of simple indices in lieu of more complex measurements of quality may be justified by demonstrating high correlations among the various measures. The confidence one may have in the index is greatly increased if the correlations observed are shown to rest on causal relationships. Furthermore, each index can be a measure of a dimension or ingredient of care. Judiciously selected multiple indices may, therefore, constitute the equivalent of borings in a geological survey which yield sufficient information about the parts to permit reconstruction of the whole. The validity of inferences about the whole will depend, of course, on the extent of internal continuities in the individual or institutional practice of medicine.

Integrative Appraisal of Quality

Most assessments of the quality of care have confined themselves to a single segment of care, almost always in the hospital. Often this segment has not even included all the care for a single episode of illness. Portions of care that precede hospitalization, and others that follow it, have been excluded. There are, thus, no well-formulated methods for evaluating care on the basis of completed episodes or for the more difficult integrative evaluation of longer sequences of care comprising many episodes. Instead we have the evaluation of what might be considered fragments of care, which, though they may sometimes be rather large, are fragments nonetheless. The evaluation of care has also been fragmented in another way: through focusing on physician care and excluding, for the most part, the contributions of all the other health professionals who constitute the totality of care. When nonphysicians have developed their own assessments, as in nursing, for example, the methods used have almost always excluded the contribution of physicans and other professions.[144, 145] Some of the reasons for this two-way fragmentation are organizational and related to such matters as the locus of responsibility for quality, the distribution of power within the medical care system and control over access to information. These matters will be described in a subsequent section of this volume. Other reasons are methodological, and will be discussed briefly here.

Several problems related to methods make it difficult to evaluate, in an integrated way, multiple segments of care. The first problem is the inadequate nature of the recorded information in most settings outside the hospital (and even in many hospitals). More complete and more uniformly standardized medical records are needed to carry out operational assessments. The fact that the poverty of records is itself related to lack of organization shows that the organizational and methodological problems merge at some points. Another problem that falls in this area of overlap is cost. Slee has pointed out that although the cost of a statistical display and analysis system, such as PAS, is a very small proportion of the cost per hospital stay, it could be a significant portion of the cost of an office visit or an episode of office care (Reference 6, page 143).

Another problem is the difficulty of determining at what intervals office care should be evaluated. Every hospital discharge provides a clear-cut end point at which the hospital stay can be evaluated as a unit. In office or clinic practice, a sequence of care may cover an indeterminate number of visits, so that identification of the appropriate unit is open to question. Usually the answer has been to choose an arbitrary time period to define the relevant episode of care. Ciocco et al. defined this as the first visit plus 14 days of follow-up.[146] Huntley et al. used a four-week period after the initial workup. Shindell has suggested that there might be a check after the first outpatient visit for each patient and subsequent ones either quarterly or semiannually (Reference 6, page 145). Solon et al. have developed, both as a concept and as an operational tool, the more rigorous notion of "episodes of medical care" for purposes of retrospective analysis.[147] This approach is a useful one and needs to be developed further. One might also consider placing upon the physician, in any given system of assessment, the responsibility of indicating when, in his opinion, an episode of care ends. The physician, using certain guidelines, would control the signals that initiate the periodic insertion of information into the system.

This discussion indicates that although the problems of evaluating the ambulatory segments of care are significant, they are by no means insurmountable where methods are concerned. This conclusion is supported by the many studies of ambulatory care referred to in previous sections of this volume. These include the studies of general practice by Peterson et al.[11] and others,[101,102] the study of the office practice of New York internists,[104] the studies of the Health Insurance Plan of Greater New York,[36,37,40,137] the early study of medical groups by Ciocco et al.[146] and the more recent study of outpatient clinic care by Huntley et al.[129]

Organizational barriers to integrative evaluation are somewhat more unyielding than the barriers of method, but even the former are giving way as organized programs of care become a more visible feature of the medical care landscape.

The conceptual and methodological problems of extending the evaluation of care to include the contributions of other professions

97

INTEGRATIVE APPRAISAL

are of a much higher order of difficulty than are those of integrating the evaluation of episodes of care; and the available **armamentarium** is currently quite meager. Much more work needs to be done in this area. We have already drawn attention to the integrative nature of end results. However, the mere examination of end results as indicators of the total impact of all the elements and strands of care is not sufficient. One needs to know the contributions of the various elements and strands. Moreover, as attention centers on the contributions of the several health professions in addition to medicine, the range of end results that are relevant, and therefore subject to assessment, is likely to be considerably broadened.

Part IV:

ISSUES OF POLICY AND IMPLEMENTATION

As he contemplates the initiation, or the expansion, of activities to assess and supervise the quality of medical care, the administrator faces issues that range from the broadest aspects of policy to the minutiae of implementation. We have already discussed some of the considerations that set the general framework for the administrative assessment of quality, described the major approaches and methods, and considered in some detail the issues that pertain to the methods and techniques of assessment. We must now consider those issues of policy and implementation that may spell success or failure in the institution of continuing quality appraisal. In so doing, we must first return to where this volume began: the general framework within which the activities of appraisal are to operate.

Objectives of Appraisal

The administrator needs to define rather clearly the general objectives of the program as well as the more specific objectives of quality review. These objectives determine not only what methods of quality review are selected, and how they are run, but also whether they are relevant or viable given the governing orientations within a particular program.

Some of the more general issues that pertain to program objectives have been discussed in the introductory section to this volume, the most important being the clear definition of the nature of responsibility assumed by the agency. First, does the agency assume responsibility for the quality of care which it provides or finances? If some responsibility for quality is undertaken, is it defined in terms of the health and welfare of a specifiable population, the overall care of a relatively stable clientele, or only in terms of those portions of care provided or purchased by the agency itself? As we have already shown, the answers to these questions determine how much emphasis is to be placed on measuring access to care, whether the favored approach is to be appraisal of outcome or of process and, if process is favored, whether segmented or integrated appraisal will be appropriate.

Having determined the scope and level of concern for quality, the next question is to determine how broadly or narrowly quality is to

APPRAISAL OBJECTIVES

be defined. Are the concerns mainly technical, or do they embrace the interpersonal and social dimensions of care? To what extent is the emphasis on discovering wasteful use, and how much concern is there for inappropriately low levels of utilization?

There is a more proximate level in the definition of objectives that relates more specifically to the most appropriate methods and techniques of assessment and to the degree of precision and rigor in those techniques. To recapitulate the discussion of these issues found in the section on Methods and Techniques: Is the primary purpose of assessment surveillance and control, research, or a combination of the two? What generalizations, if any, are to be made on the basis of the data? The answers to such questions determine, as we have already described, the nature of the samples to be drawn, the manner in which the standards are formulated and applied, and the degree of rigor and precision called for in the methods of measurement and the construction of scales. The sophistication of method required to separate out a group in which there is a high probability of care being bad is certainly very different from that required to place care and/or providers precisely at some point along an extended scale (Cecil Sheps in Reference 6, page 34).

The administrator must also determine the proper balance between the educational objectives of quality assessment and the need to deter and detect careless or incompetent practice. There is general agreement that the purpose should be primarily to contribute to the continuing self-examination and education of the medical staff. However, there is also a responsibility to protect the patient, the care-providing institution, and the third party payer against any physicians who are either ill-qualified for what they attempt to provide or unscrupulous in the conduct of their practice. The question faced by the administrator is how to set the proper balance between the two objectives of education and discipline.

In real life, the answer appears to depend in part on the role and influence of the practicing physicians on the program. Wherever this influence is small, as in some health insurance programs, there is either no responsibility for quality or, at best, emphasis is placed on the identification and correction of abuse that borders on the criminal. Wherever the role of the practicing physician is significantly large, or dominant, the emphasis may fall so predominantly on the educational objective that the disciplinary objective is in danger of being ignored or explicitly excluded. Many factors account for this imbalance. Fundamentally, the control of behavior within the medical profession is brought about not by the coercive power of superior authority, but by the operation of ethical standards that prescribe responsibility to patients and sensitivity to the good opinion of colleagues. This fundamental orientation is reinforced by notions concerning the nature and frequency of deviations from accepted practice and what accounts for them. It is asserted that most physicians are motivated to provide good care and to use the hospital in an appropriate manner. Deviations are believed to be caused by occasional inattention, by gradual, unintentional drift into bad habits or technical obsolescence, or by pervasive administrative and organizational constraints over which the physician has little control. Flagrant abuse is said to be a rare phenomenon. As a consequence, significant improvements in the levels of care, and savings in hospital days inappropriately used, are not likely to be achieved by detecting and correcting abuse, but by bringing about smaller, and more pervasive, changes in the practice of a much larger number of physicians. It is the cumulative effect of these smaller adjustments, influencing the mass of physicians, that is expected to pay the greatest dividends. Finally, any approach that leads to the exclusion or elimination of specified physicians from program participation is considered to be socially undesirable because it simply permits the physician to continue practice in the general community, unsupported and unsupervised (Payne in Reference 6, page 38).

Empirical evidence in support of these viewpoints is not easy to come by. Goss has documented the nonbureaucratic nature of colleague relationships in a hospital outpatient clinic.[148] Freidson and Rhea have shown the weaknesses of formal and informal organizational control on physician behavior in a prepaid group practice and suggested that a major avenue to bringing about acceptable behavior is to recruit physicians responsive to the standards and norms of the group.[103] The performance of general practitioners under observation seems to support the contention that confirmed habits and technical obsolescence are major factors in poor performance.[11, 101] As already mentioned, Shindell has reported that inappropriate hospital use represents pervasive intrahospital behavior rather than significantly deviant behavior on the part of a small number of individuals.[25, 30, 31] On the other hand, Lembcke has reported a relatively precipitous, eightfold reduction in the performance of criticized gynecological operations in one hospital when it became known that an external audit was in progress.[41] This suggests that physicians are aware of deficiencies in their own practice and that they respond to the threat of external supervision. Further findings will be described in a subsequent section on the effectiveness of methods of quality and utilization appraisal.

Certain important consequences flow from a predominant emphasis

APPRAISAL OBJECTIVES

on the educational purposes of quality appraisal. It would seem that this emphasis is more in keeping with the institution of internal, rather than external, audits. The external audit must be handled with great care if it is to be seen as educational rather than punitive. There should be careful initial preparation to ensure cooperative participation. The results of the audit must be thoroughly discussed with the physicians involved. Such discussion cannot be limited to the presentation of statistical findings that are either poorly understood or considered to be inconclusive. As Morehead has emphasized, the presentation of concrete clinical examples is essential to successful communication and to bringing about change.[40]

The emphasis on the educational mission of quality appraisal would also seem to support those who advocate participation by the hospital medical staff in formulating the audit standards so that there is knowledge of what the standards are and agreement concerning their applicability. The educational objective does not prescribe, however, that the standards must be entirely local, since these may simply perpetuate pervasive local error. The most helpful approach may be a combination of externally determined normative standards with adaptation to local use, as advocated by Payne.[47] Alternatively, there may be comparisons of practice among local institutions, as advocated by Shindell,[30-32] combined with the more general comparisons made possible by a system of national scope such as PAS.[27, 28]

When the emphasis is exclusively on education and the achievement of organizational change, there is a reluctance to identify any individual whose performance deviates from the average or the norm. This phenomenon is clearly seen in the activities of the Hospital Utilization Project (HUP) as described by Shindell.[30-32] Here the emphasis is on identifying the patterns of usual practice with respect to the most frequent diagnoses, on the "profiles" of each hospital with respect to the diagnoses under study, and on the position of each hospital with respect to other hospitals. While hospitals are identified and ranked, physicians seldom are. Payne exercises and recommends the same restraint in the application of the "criteria approach":

> In reporting the cases . . . to the staff, we never individualized as to physicians. And I think this is important, because, if this is to be the educational effort that we want it to be, we cannot single out a physician, and say, "You're wearing the black hat, and the other guy is wearing the white hat." They will know from their own performance as related to reported incidents of omissions or commissions in the report. And their responsiveness is to me the evidence that this is an effective approach (Reference 6, page 238).

The decision not to individualize must appeal not only to physicians, but also to administrators faced with ensuring acceptability for quality appraisal and fearful of medical opposition. However, total unwillingness to identify and deal individually with deviant cases appears to run counter to practice already current in tissue and audit committees in many hospitals. It is not in keeping with case-by-case certification and review procedures such as those called for by Medicare [15] or instituted by the New Jersey Blue Cross in cooperation with physicians and hospitals. A more reasonable approach would be to combine, in a manner that appears most feasible and productive to the administrator, the concern for general patterns of care with the need to detect and deal with significant deviance from such patterns. The two approaches would seem to be mutually supportive rather than antithetical, provided they are carried out with discretion and good judgment.

Another issue, relating partly to objectives and partly to methods and techniques, is the distinction between the preventive and interventive approaches to the assessment of quality and utilization. As Donabedian has pointed out, the usual processes of review are retrospective rather than concurrent, and provide no opportunity for intervention during the course of any one episode of care.[5] This can be a major weakness. A program, such as Workmen's Compensation, that provides or finances medical care may need frequent feedback concerning the status of persons under care, and may require the power to intervene when it becomes apparent that the provider is unqualified to carry out what he proposes to do, or when there is good reason to believe that care is inappropriate, inadequate or excessive. Although the notion of intervention is certain to run counter to established professional traditions, it nevertheless requires serious consideration in setting up any procedure of formal review. Such intervention apparently is practiced in the Ontario Workmen's Compensation program.[149] It is clearly envisaged in proposals made by the Committee on Trauma of the American College of Surgeons. To quote from this remarkable document:

> In cases where the medical director believes that medical care may not be competent or when in his opinion recovery has not been satisfactory or has been unduly delayed, he should have the right to an examination not only of the patient, but also of all physicians' and hospital records, including laboratory findings and X-ray films. Such examinations may be made by the director himself or at his discretion by panels of impartial medically qualified experts or their designees. . . . In cases where incompetent or inadequate medical care is corroborated by the panel, the medical director may then transfer the patient to a qualified expert designated by the panel for further treatment.[150]

APPRAISAL RESPONSIBILITY

As already pointed out, the AID system of variable-interval certification provides an opportunity for concurrent review. It is, fundamentally, an interventive approach even though the major responsibility for intervention is delegated to the managing physician himself. With the development of on line, real time computer systems, it should be possible to achieve a significantly greater capacity for concurrent appraisal. Whether this methodological refinement is linked with intervention or not becomes a matter of policy. In any event, it is an area for further thought and research.

Finally, the perspective of the agency—whether it is long term or short term—will influence the emphasis on approaches to appraisal. Shapiro has pointed out that many end result studies are directed to program improvement over the long haul rather than to immediate controls over the management of cases (Reference 6, page 111).

Responsibility for Appraisal

Social concern—its nature, degree and location—for the quality of professional performance is undoubtedly the single most important factor that influences the initiation of quality appraisal, the choice of methods for carrying it out and the prospects for its viability and effectiveness.

The quality of medical care has always been a matter of social concern. However, such concern, in the past, seems to have been delegated almost entirely to professional organizations and institutions with specific legal, and more general social, support. Traditionally, the medical profession has discharged its responsibilities for quality by (1) controlling entry into the profession; (2) controlling education and training so as to assure the acquisition of knowledge and skill and the internalization of appropriate values; (3) confirming the competence of the finished product through licensure and certification; and, to a lesser degree, (4) providing opportunities for continuing education and renewal. The control of quality through formal supervision and review is a fairly recent, and relatively foreign, element in professional life.

Nevertheless, the profession in general, and professional organizations in particular, have in recent years paid increasing attention to the institution and nurturance of mechanisms that permit physicians to evaluate and correct their own work. Notable among these is the early work of the American College of Surgeons that led to the establishment of the Joint Commission on Accreditation of Hospitals with its dominant emphasis on the self-governing, self-evaluating activities of the organized hospital medical staff.[151] In general, the rise of specialization, and of organizations of specialists, has created a cadre of physicians more sensitive to standards of performance, and more determined that special competence be appropriately recognized and rewarded.

As indicated in the appropriate sections, several of the methods described in the present volume owe their inception and success to support by professional organizations. These methods include the New Jersey AID certification system,[22–24] the statistical display and analysis systems as developed by the Commission on Professional and Hospital Activities[27–29] and the Hospital Utilization Project.[30–32] Moreover, we have referred in this volume to publications that demonstrate interest in, or support for, various methods of utilization review by the American Medical Association[44] and state medical societies in California,[117] Pennsylvania[118] and New York.[113] The American Medical Association has published a description of professional review mechanisms in which the organized profession has played a major role.[152]

The reader must realize, however, that professional encouragement and support for the appraisal of quality and utilization is provided under certain conditions. First, the processes of appraisal and correction are envisaged to be under exclusive or predominant professional control and, second, the appraisal of utilization is more readily acceptable than the appraisal of aspects of quality which involve the more technical elements of professional judgment. The administrator must also be prepared to find, in any particular local situation, powerful elements of the conservative tradition that opposes the relatively recent phenomenon of quality appraisal and surveillance.

Certain developments have intensified social concern for quality, brought about changes in the location of responsibility for assuring its achievement, and opened the way for increasing emphasis on continuing review of professional performance as a mechanism of quality control.

Primarily in response to technological imperatives, medical practice has been conducted, to an increasing degree, in organized settings such as the hospital or a group practice, where professional behavior is subject to observation by professional colleagues. Moreover, the nature of social and legal corporate responsibility for quality is being redefined. Increasingly, the hospital is being vested with responsibility for the care provided by the seemingly independent private practitioners who constitute its staff.[153]

With the increasing organization of practice, sweeping changes have occurred in the organization of financing and provision of care.

APPRAISAL RESPONSIBILITY

So-called "third parties"—insurance agencies, government programs, organized labor and industry—are all concerned with the quantity and quality of care which they help to purchase or provide. As medical care becomes more publicly important, it becomes less an exclusive professional preserve, and increasingly an arena where diverse interests clamor to be heard.

The play of these forces is well illustrated by the active role played by hospital associations, as well as Blue Cross and Blue Shield agencies, in the support of the mechanisms of review described in this volume. The inception of the New Jersey system of variable-interval certification (AID) illustrates more clearly than usual the effect of widespread concern about rising hospital costs and the chain of events that bring about the institution of intraprofessional surveillance:

> The rising average length of stay . . . the constant per diem rise of hospital costs . . . and resultant necessity for rate increase applications by Blue Cross to the New Jersey State Department of Banking and Insurance—all these factors culminated into a demand for stronger measures to contain increased, improper or unnecessary hospital utilization . . . (Reference 23, pages 2–3).

> Fortunately, or unfortunately, we were stimulated to a great extent by the Commissioner of Banking and Insurance who regulates us, and he indicated to the medical society and the New Jersey Hospital Association, not Blue Cross or Blue Shield, that they've got to do something in order to eliminate unnecessary stay . . . (Reference 25, page 68).

> The State Commissioner of Banking and Insurance . . . issued a strong endorsement of the program referring to it as a "potentially powerful" step in the effort to stabilize Blue Cross and Blue Shield rates, and urging the full cooperation of hospitals, doctors and patients in implementing the program to assure its success. A similar endorsement was issued by the executive board of the New Jersey Industrial Union Council, AFL-CIO . . . (Reference 22, page 4).

In any medical care program, the decision to institute a process of review, as well as the form and content of the review, depend on the function assigned to the responsible agency, the manner in which the agency views its responsibility, and its willingness or ability to exercise the requisite degree of influence or control. There is little doubt that any agency engaged in the direct provision of care, through its own facilities and staff, should be responsible for the quality of care that it provides. There is less acceptance of the principle that an agency, government or private, which merely finances medical care services has a similar responsibility to assure the quality of care it helps to purchase. This principle has been traditionally neglected by insurance agencies, and government programs have varied greatly with regard to it. The problem has been especially acute in public welfare medical care where, in addition to the usual governmental reluctance to assume responsibility for quality, there has been the public policy question of whether the indigent should have better medical care than that currently available to the bulk of the self-supporting.

Donabedian has summarized the reasons which, in his opinion, furnish convincing argument for the assumption of program responsibility by the financing agency for the quality of care.[154, 155] These are: (1) deficiencies in the prevailing levels of quality, (2) inability of the consumer to judge the technical dimensions of quality, (3) the rather narrow definition of quality by some providers, (4) limitations in self-defined standards of quality, (5) the effects of organization on quality, even when such effects are unintended, and (6) the availability of mechanisms which offer reasonable assurance that quality can be improved by specific administrative action.

If the quality of medical care were of the highest, in all situations and places, there would be much less need for the agency to be concerned. Although there are no studies of national scope on the basis of which one can generalize concerning the quality of care, the examination of certain end results, such as infant mortality in this country compared with others, does not justify optimism or complacency. In recent years, the reduction of U. S. infant mortality was achieved to a lesser extent than in 14 other "advanced countries." In 1960–61, nine of these countries had lower infant mortality rates than the United States, signifying a relative worsening in our position during the previous decade.[156] In fact, "Not one of the U. S. States had infant death rates in 1962 as low as the 15.3 per 1,000 in the Netherlands and Sweden, but ranged from the low of 19.7 in Utah to 40 in Mississippi. If all the States had rates as low as in Utah, the lives of 23,000 who now die before their first birthday would be spared."[157] Infant mortality has been an especially serious problem in the larger cities.[156] ". . . Only Houston and Los Angeles among the 10 largest cities had lower infant deaths in 1961 than in 1950. In all but four of these cities (New York, Los Angeles, Houston, and the District of Columbia) the death rate increased for white as well as for nonwhite infants during this period."[157] During 1950–1954, the relative contribution of component segments of infant mortality in some census tracts of Metropolitan Boston was similar to that of the United States as a whole in 1915, and comparable with the current pattern in partially developed countries. "With respect to infant mortality, some areas of a modern American metropolis appear to be four decades behind the times."[158] It is recognized, of course, that factors other than medical care influence infant mortality, and might account, in part, for differences among nations.[159] However, it is likely that inadequacies in the quantity and quality of medical care play a significant role in bringing about such end results as those described.

The study of the medical care process provides more direct information, although this is not of national scope. Nevertheless, whenever the quality of care has been studied in specific situations, serious deficiencies have come to light. The following are examples culled from the literature of the last two decades: In North Carolina, 44 percent of general practitioners were found to practice at levels described as below average or poor. In most instances the deficiencies were gross and unquestionable.[11] In a study of perinatal mortality in New York City, 42 percent of deaths in mature infants and 29 percent of deaths in premature infants were judged to have been preventable, at least in part. Errors of medical judgment or technique were noted in many of these.[84] In a study of hysterectomies performed in 35 privately administered hospitals in the Los Angeles Area 60 percent of operations were judged to have been justified, 28 percent probably not justified and 12 percent not justified.[160] Lembcke has reported that about 70 percent of castrating gynecological operations in one hospital were criticized as a result of an external audit.[41]

When the management of selected diagnostic categories was assessed in one hospital in the Boston Metropolitan area, 28 percent of medical cases, 35 percent of surgical cases and 50 percent of cases in the category of obstetrics and gynecology were rated as poor.[100] The management of hospitalized illness for families of workers belonging to the Teamsters Union in New York City was judged to have been fair or poor in a little over 40 percent of the cases.[38, 39] To some degree, defects in quality persist even under the most prestigious of auspices. In St. Luke's Hospital, New York City, as many as 90 percent of operative deaths in children and infants were judged to have been preventable.[85] In the outpatient department of a teaching hospital, routine procedures were not carried out in 15 percent of cases, and abnormalities that were found were not followed in 22 percent of cases.[129] The clear conclusion to be drawn is that quality cannot be taken for granted. It needs to be planned for and watched over.

A very significant feature of the findings on prevalent levels of quality is the wide range in the quality of performance encountered among hospitals and physicians. The study, by Doyle, of hysterectomies in Los Angeles hospitals showed that the percent of cases not justified and probably not justified ranged from 5 percent in one hospital to 84 percent in another. Eisele *et al.* showed similarly wide divergences in practice among 15 general hospitals and their physicians.[35] Some of their findings are summarized in Tabulation IV-1:

Tabulation IV-1.

| | Percent of Cases Cared for in Each Category ||
Categories of Care	Hospitals	Physicians with 10 Cases or More in Each Category
Primary appendectomies not justified by finding of acute appendicitis in the surgical specimen	32–82	13–100
Diagnosis of diabetes without a record of blood sugar determination	5–55	4–100*
Diagnosis of diabetes without record of chest X-ray	54–96	—
Chest X-ray not taken in cases with acute lower respiratory infection	5–55	0–75*

* Value estimated from graph.

Tabulation IV-2 presents somewhat more recent data, also based on information assembled by the Commission on Professional and Hospital Activities, and shows the following ranges among five general hospitals: [161]

Tabulation IV-2.

Operations	Percent of Operations Not Justified by Tissue Disease
All operations	14–37%
Operations on uterus	12–59
Gastrectomy	22–44
Operations on tubes and/or ovaries	15–41
Simple mastectomy	7–40
Operations on thyroid	1–36
Appendectomy	15–35
Cholecystectomy	0–18

Additional data, of a similar nature, will be cited below. It is clear that we must face squarely the question of why one hospital should find an achievement possible, whereas another doesn't, and of why one physician's accomplishments should be so different from another's.

The responsibility of the administrator, and of the institution or organized program of medical care which he represents, becomes even more critical because the consumer is usually unable to judge for himself the technical aspects of the quality of the medical care which he receives. This contention is supported by anecdotal experience.[162] It is more formally documented in a study in which the judgments of expert assessors were compared with the opinions of those who received the care in question.[38] For cases in which care was judged to have been excellent or good, 86 percent of patients expressed the opinion that they had received the "best" care. For cases judged by experts to have been fair or poor, 74 percent of patients felt they had received the best care. At the same time, in the second category of cases only five percent of patients said the care received had been "not good." Other studies also support the contention that the consumer is ill equipped to assess the technical quality of care. The North Carolina study of general practice showed that the busiest physicians were not necessarily the best. Studies made by the Health Insurance Plan of Greater New York have shown that, within group practice, some of the poorest physicians have many patients who are very happy with the care they receive. Some of the groups that have the fewest complaints from their patients show up less well on measurements of quality than groups having more complaints. When the consumer can be so ill equipped to protect his own interests, society is called upon to remedy the defect.

A third reason for the exercise of program responsibility is the narrow, technical orientation that many physicians seem to exhibit in the conduct of their practice. Preventive, anticipatory and rehabilitative management are said to have very low priority, and some aspects of interpersonal and social management are virtually ignored. While most authorities in medical care organization would support these impressions, there is little actual research to confirm them. One study that appears to do so is a survey of physicians named by a representative sample of the adult U. S. population in 1955 as their "regular doctor" or the doctor they would "probably call" if they got sick.[163] When asked about specified diagnostic procedures that should be routinely performed annually for all adults, the physicians responded as follows: checkups even if person feels well, 74 percent; rectal examination, 68 percent; pelvic examination, 76 percent; chest X-rays for men over 45, 77 percent. It appears that action at the program level may be necessary to bring about implementation in practice of newer and broader concepts of the quality of care.

The program may also need to exercise responsibility because physicians in the solo practice of medicine, especially those who have a relatively inactive hospital practice, tend to suffer from professional isolation and lose the ability to be critical of their own work. This is also likely to be true in certain hospitals where an ingrown group of physicians tends to become unwarrantably satisfied with the work they do collectively. It is necessary to confront such "closed systems" of self-satisfaction or mutual admiration with the harsher realities of external standards.

The fact that any system for the organized delivery of care, by virtue of its very existence and the features of its program and organization, must influence the patterns and quality of care, places a heavy responsibility on the program in question. There is no room in this volume to review the studies that have concerned themselves with the relationships between the manner in which a program is organized and the quality of care which it provides. The studies of Morehead et al. may be cited as an illustration of the kinds of factors involved and of the interactions among these factors.

Table 3 shows the relationships between certain hospital character-

Table 3. Percent of Hospital Admissions Judged To Have Received "Less than Optimal" Care, by Accreditation Status and Type of Hospital.*

Type of Hospital	Accredited	Not Accredited
Voluntary, affiliated with medical school	14	—
Voluntary, not affiliated with a medical school, but approved for training of interns, residents or both	45	—
Voluntary, not affiliated with a medical school and having no approved training programs	47	60
Proprietary Hospitals	57	52

* Teamster Family Members, New York City, Circa 1962.
Source: M. A. Morehead. Personal communication based on data from Morehead et al., Reference 39.

istics and quality ratings arrived at by record review. It is clear that the largest differences in levels of quality exist between hospitals affiliated with medical schools and those that have no such affiliation. It is equally clear that accreditation, in and of itself, may not be an important factor in safeguarding quality in some situations. Table 4 shows the interaction of the effects of physician qualifications and hospital characteristics on the quality of hospital care as judged by record review. In both affiliated hospitals and nonproprietary hospitals not affiliated with a medical school, whether or not a physician is a specialty board diplomate does not appear to be related to quality. The characteristics of the hospital, presumably achieved by the manner in which it selects and directs its medical staff, rather than by the formal qualifications of the staff, appear to be the key factor. In proprietary hospitals, where the organizational factors are less powerful and more variable, the formal qualifications of the medical practitioners emerge as a strong factor in relation to quality of care provided. The physician without specialist qualifications and with-

Table 4. **Percent of Hospital Admissions Judged To Have Received "Less than Optimal" Care by Type of Hospital and by Physician Qualification.***

	Physician Qualifications		
Type of Hospital	Diplomate or Fellow†	Appointment at Municipal or Voluntary Hospital‡	Privileges at Proprietary Hospital Only§
Affiliated with medical school	14	6	—
Not affiliated with medical school	46	54	—
Proprietary	30	56	71

* Teamster Family Members, New York City, Circa 1962.
† Diplomate of American Specialty Board or Fellow of an American college.
‡ Not Diplomate or Fellow, but with municipal or voluntary hospital appointment.
§ Not Diplomate or Fellow and with no appointment at a municipal or voluntary hospital.
Source: Morehead et al., Reference 39.

out an appointment at a voluntary or municipal hospital is especially likely to be guilty of poor practice. As many as 71 percent of cases cared for by such physicians were judged to have received less than optimal care.

The sensitivity of medical practice to certain organizational factors is elegantly demonstrated by a study of "unnecessary" appendectomies in Baltimore hospitals.[164] Table 5 presents the essential data. In

Table 5. **Percent of Primary Appendectomies Classified Pathologically as "Unnecessary" or "Doubtful" in Two University and Three Community Hospitals by Type of Hospital and Patient Pay Status.***

	Hospital	
Pay Status of Patients	University Hospitals	Community Hospitals
Welfare (N=96)	33	40
Private pay (N=186)	35	42
Insurance other than Blue Cross (N=165)	35	50
Blue Cross (N=555)	34	55

* Baltimore, 1957 and 1958.
Source: Reference 164.
Note: The percentages in this table have been estimated from Figure 2 in the original paper. Information concerning the number of cases in each cell is not available. There were 404 cases in the university hospitals and 598 cases in the community hospitals.

teaching hospitals, the percent of such appendectomies is lower than in other community hospitals. Moreover, in teaching hospitals the percent of "unnecessary" appendectomies is not related to the patient's pay status. In the community hospitals, on the other hand, "unnecessary" appendectomies are not only proportionately more frequent, but are also related to the pay status of the patient in a remarkably regular manner.

Finally, program responsibility for the quality of care is increased by the availability of reasonably effective mechanisms for quality appraisal and surveillance. These include the methods to which this volume has been devoted. Evidence concerning the effectiveness of these methods will be cited below.

Since the quality of medical care provided is dependent on how the hospital (or program) is organized and on the presence (or absence) within it of appropriate mechanisms of quality surveillance, the administrator cannot evade the social responsibility for quality. Even if he decides to ignore this responsibility, what he does, or fails to do, is often reflected in the quality of care that the institution or program provides. Briefly, the responsibility for quality can be ignored but not evaded!

The administrator in a public or quasi-public program appears to be under a special obligation, where quality is concerned, since it is the expected role of such agencies to guard the general interest in a manner that transcends particular or sectional interests.

Whether for the reasons cited above, or for others, public and quasi-public agencies have increasingly accepted some responsibility for quality. Medicare, in spite of the disclaimer that nothing in the act shall mean supervision or control over the practice of medicine or the manner in which medical services are provided,[165] has signified that quality is a central concern by setting up explicit conditions for institutional participation and by establishing procedures to review professional care. The utilization review procedures clearly encompass the appropriateness of service and, hence, the quality of medical care.[15] We thus have not only public approval, but public requirement that the process of care be brought under continuing scrutiny. This orientation is likely to have a profound influence on other private and public programs, as is already apparent in the Federal regulations for the Medicaid program. Some localities and states have moved even further, as is witnessed by regulations governing Medicaid in New York City and State.[166-168] Other examples of more demanding governmental standards are those for the amputees' program, and for proprietary nursing homes in New York City.[169, 170] Even more inclusive is legislation enacted in New York State that provides for "the establishment of requirements for a uniform state-

APPRAISAL RESPONSIBILITY

wide system of reports and audits relating to the quality of medical care provided, hospital utilization and costs" in all hospitals.[171] The development of methods and procedures for statewide hospital audits is now in progress.[172]

An important question to consider is how to delegate the responsibility for the quality of medical care—how much should be retained and exercised directly? How much responsibility should be consigned to another agency or to the practicing physicians themselves? For example, to what extent should a health insurance program, whether governmental, quasi-public or private, be directly involved in appraisal of care, and to what extent may it rely on the participating hospitals, the organized staff within the hospital, or the local medical society to carry out the function of appraisal and supervision? The general tendency is for such "third parties" to rely upon the care-providing institutions and physicians for the supervision of care. An excellent example of this is Medicare. In this instance, the Social Security Administration demands assurances that certain mechanisms for the review of the appropriateness of care have been instituted and are in operation.[15] It does not, itself, conduct independent studies of the quality of care to verify the performance of the intrainstitutional review bodies.

There are exceptions to the preference for delegation of the appraisal function. The Health Insurance Plan of Greater New York has assumed the obligation, and the right, to assess independently the quality of care provided by the autonomous medical groups that contract to provide care for Plan subscribers. The studies of quality already referred to are the result of this arrangement.[36, 37, 40, 137] These are, in effect, external audits conducted by the financing organization, and are additional to any quality appraisal and control mechanisms enforced internally by the groups themselves. Situations where public agencies have assumed a similar role of external auditor include the surveillance exercised over perinatal deaths by the Chicago Health Department,[83] and the much more ambitious external audits of hospital care prescribed by law, and in process of development, in New York State.[171, 172]

Even in those situations in which the financing agency appears to have delegated the function of appraisal to the providers of care, the delegation is usually not complete. There is some provision for an independent check on use of service and, sometimes, on the quality of care. We have already referred to the systems of claim verification and utilization review in insurance programs.[17, 113] Medicare has available to it information which will permit constant surveillance of patterns of care at the aggregate level.[173] This should provide intelligence concerning the state of the system as a whole, and reveal whether the delegation of appraisal and control activities has proven to be successful.[174]

The variable-interval certification system (AID) provides an interesting example of delegation with provision for verification at two successive levels. As we have already described, the managing physician himself makes the initial decision concerning appropriateness of stay within the framework of established standards of length of stay. His decision to extend stay beyond the prescribed period of time is subject to review both by a committee of his peers within the hospital and by the Blue Cross agency, which can act independently to bring to the attention of the hospital utilization review committee questionable features of the physician's practice.[22]

The administrator must, in each instance, decide to what extent the appraisal function is to be delegated, and to what extent it is to be retained by the central agency. Delegation of this function to well-organized institutions and groups of physicians capable of carrying out the necessary activities has many obvious advantages.[26] Unfortunately, as we shall describe in the next section, there are significant obstacles to the successful implementation of quality review functions by providers. Therefore, the central agency must institute a system of independent checks to assure itself that the peripheral system of appraisal, at the provider level, is in good repair. What these checks are depends, in part, on the scope of the program and its resources. Ideally, the program should contain all of the following components: (1) a method for finding out whether the appraisal mechanisms promised by the providers are in actual existence and operation; (2) a method for replicating, on a sample basis, the activities of the appraisal mechanisms instituted by the providers; and (3) a system that monitors selected medical care activities and outcomes so as to provide an indication of the state of the program as a whole.

One aspect of the responsibility for the quality of care is the innovating and enabling role played by professional organizations and their allied insurance agencies. Effects of this kind of happy collaboration can be traced in the development, and present operations, of the Commission on Professional and Hospital Activities (CPHA), the Hospital Utilization Project (HUP), and other programs in which organized medicine and health insurance have worked together.[152] Shindell has remarked:

> In Western Pennsylvania, utilization efforts preceded Medicare by about five years and were developed because a sense of responsibility was felt by many members of organized medicine locally . . . the Project is a voluntary effort undertaken by the medical profession and hospital association of a community, with aid from the principal health insurer, to provide a service to the utilization committees of the hospitals in that community. The

service consists of the furnishing of comparative data to reflect length of stay experience within the community as well as technical assistance in dealing with the possible problems revealed by the data (Reference 30, pages 1 and 2).

Both CPHA and HUP have played an important role in developing techniques for data display and analysis. They have used these techniques to provide information concerning quality of care and the factors that influence it. They have also made possible the wider application of these techniques through education as well as through more direct forms of assistance. Such activities illustrate the central agency's responsibility to assist the care-providing agencies in the conduct of quality appraisal and supervision.

Implementation

The implementation of quality appraisal and utilization review rests on several conditions: (1) the organization of practice, (2) the assumption of responsibility for quality, (3) acceptability to physicians, and (4) acceptability to the administrator. The central role of the assumption of responsibility has been discussed. The remaining conditions listed will be discussed below.

Organization of practice includes the structuring of (a) the profession itself into local, state, and national associations, (b) financing through health insurance or tax-supported programs, (c) the conduct of care by private practitioners in organized settings such as the hospital, and (d) the delivery of care itself through the employment of full-time staff. This list indicates a rough progression to higher levels of organization and an increasing potential for quality appraisal and supervision. Organization localizes and makes visible the responsibility both for quality and for the financial impact of inappropriate and wasteful use. Furthermore, it provides the enabling mechanisms and the power leverage necessary to gain access to information concerning care and to bring about the participation of physicians in the processes of self-examination and self-correction.

In a pluralistic medical care system, such as ours, the implementation of quality and utilization appraisal often requires cooperation and accommodation among several power groups: organized medicine, quasi-public and private health insurance, the hospitals and their associations, and government. Examples of such collaboration have already been cited. We have emphasized the responsibility of "third parties" for quality, as well as their potential to provide financial resources, technical equipment and know-how. Densen has emphasized the need for government either to be directly involved or to support mechanisms outside government for administrative quality appraisal and basic research in the quality of care (Reference 6, page 103). He has also pointed out the opportunities within the Medicare program for the development of such mechanisms and research activities (Reference 6, pages 108–110).

A primary condition for the implementation of quality appraisal and utilization review is acceptability of such procedures to the physicians involved, and their informed collaboration. If these are not secured, the administrator is almost always faced with an insurmountable barrier to effective implementation.

> Medical staff acceptance is by far the most important hurdle. A realistic approach must recognize that many medical staffs feel any formal approach to the measurement of quality of care is a threat to their autonomy, their responsible behavior, their privileges, their independence of action, their freedom to experiment and an open invitation to malpractice suits. All these charges must be answered to insure the degree of staff participation that makes such a procedure useful to physicians (Payne in Reference 45, page 4).

Approval by professional accrediting bodies and national and local medical associations lends legitimacy to mechanisms of appraisal and review.[26] The increasing organization of practice creates settings within which these mechanisms gain acceptability. However, even within highly organized settings, the notion of quality appraisal, especially if it involves an instrumentality outside the medical staff itself, remains foreign, disquieting or downright unacceptable. Appraisal confined to the appropriateness of the use of services and resources is more palatable, especially if the concern is limited to patterns of care, and the contributions of individual physicians are not identified. Very often the shortage in hospital beds, and the consequent competition for them, has already attuned physicians to the need for some controls over utilization. Thus, certain programs, for example the Hospital Utilization Project, have been careful to confine themselves to the general patterns of hospital utilization. Of course appropriateness of use is an important element in the quality of care, and review of utilization has ramifications that touch upon the most sensitive areas of physician judgment. Nevertheless, some authorities have suggested that the institution of utilization review should be used as a planned first step in the introduction of a broader program of quality appraisal. Presumably, the progression would be, in order of acceptability, (1) review of the patterns of hospital admissions and components of length of stay, (2) expansion of the study of patterns of care to include other elements of management by diagnosis, and finally, if at all, (3) the study of individual physician performance. Other authorities have felt that this degree of caution is unnecessary, and that multidimensional quality appraisal, with or without individualization, will be found acceptable to many physicians in many communities.

Often, the exclusion of what are regarded as administrative intrusions, external agencies, and external criteria is one important condition for physician acceptance. Shindell has recounted the efforts of HUP to develop criteria for appropriate hospital use. Opposition to the use of "criteria" as a standard of practice was so intense that they were withdrawn (Reference 25, pages 48 to 49) and replaced by "Guides for Case Review" designed to insure consistency in the review of cases in selected diagnostic categories.[30a] Payne was unable to get the Michigan Medical Society's official endorsement for the Manual,[47] which lists criteria for about 50 diagnoses.

A final condition for physician acceptance is the voluntary nature of the appraisal scheme. Shindell has emphasized this feature of HUP and pointed out that with appropriate preparation, and the provision of a service of recognized value, community support and participation can be high.[30] The Commission on Professional and Hospital Activities has sold its services to over a thousand U. S. hospitals. Mikelbank has reported excellent cooperation by physicians in implementing the AID program in New Jersey.

> A study made during the four months May–August 1965 revealed that only 1500 cases had to be returned requesting a physician's certification. This represents only two percent of the total number of claims paid. Initially there were a few physicians who actually refused to complete the physician's statement when the length of stay exceeded the number of days authorized and in such cases the hospitals billed the patients. The Plan had no repercussions from the patient. From time to time "pockets of resistance" arise but they are generally overcome either through persuasion or (by) the fact that the patient is requested to pay the hospital bill beyond the number of days allowed in the AID Manual for the diagnosis for which the physician is treating the patient (Reference 23, page 7).

By contrast to the emphasis on voluntarism, Medicare incorporates legal requirements for intrainstitutional utilization review [15] and New York State has a legal requirement for external audits of hospital care.[171] Such legal enactments may simply represent somewhat belated official recognition of activities that have been developed within the profession and have gained a large measure of professional legitimacy and support.[107, 152] Under these conditions, legal recognition may provide the added impetus needed to achieve universal acceptance. However, one must face the possibility that in local situations where legitimacy is not recognized, and staff support not forthcoming, the internal review procedures required by law will be accorded only token compliance.

The reader should not infer from the above the existence of a simple dichotomy of voluntarism versus compulsion. The forces that bear upon the implementation of quality controls are far more complex. Much that appears to be voluntary in American medicine is influential almost to the point of compulsion. This includes the requirements for admission to voluntary hospital staffs, accreditation, participation in health insurance and in governmental programs such as Medicare, and responsiveness to the financial interests of patients who are entitled to benefits from such programs.

Another factor in the implementation of quality appraisal and utilization review is acceptability to the administrator. Needless to say, the program administrator has a high stake in assuring the most productive use of a limited budget. Similarly, the interest of the hospital administrator in appropriate hospital use under conditions of excessively high occupancy can well be appreciated. The incentive may be reduced, however, when the hospital is half empty.

An important selling point of statistical systems such as HUP and PAS is that they generate products which the hospital administrator would in any case need to run the hospital, to meet the requirements for accreditation, and to participate in government programs such as Medicare. Some of these products are basic patient statistics, indexes of diagnoses and operations, and information on length of stay. However, the administrator needs to be motivated by a deep sense of responsibility for the quality of care if he is to initiate and bring about meaningful quality review in the face of indifference or opposition by appreciable segments of his medical staff. In such an effort, support by key members of his staff and by the more pervasive outside forces that we have referred to, would be critical.

The administrator's role in quality appraisal and utilization review contains some ambiguity due to the general contention on the part of physicians that matters relating to medical judgment should remain the exclusive province of the physician. The clear intent of review and audit activities is to give each profession the task of supervising the performance of its own members. This does not mean, as we have pointed out, that responsibility is entirely so delegated. For example, in the hospital, the board of trustees and the administrator must see to it that the appropriate review mechanisms are set up and kept at peak performance. Furthermore, the professional health services administrator can readily review, understand and interpret to the board of trustees a large share of the data cumulated through statistical tabulation and case review. He may, in fact, be more adept at the manipulation, display and interpretation of statistical data than the clinical staff. Administrative review of professional activities is, therefore, both feasible and necessary. Although final judgment concerning the technical dimensions of quality remains within the province of professional competence, the administrator must participate actively in maintaining the apparatus of quality control. He must also participate in setting the standards for those dimensions of quality that are not exclusively technical in nature.[5]

An important component of implementation is achieving the appropriate use of the procedures for review installed in a given setting. This is often a serious problem in systems, such as HUP or PAS, to which a hospital may subscribe. The statistical displays and analyses which such systems generate are transmitted to each participating hospital and may be exhaustively used, or simply filed away and forgotten (Morehead, Reference 6, page 127; Weinerman, Reference 6, page 128). The reason for their neglect may lie partly in a lack of real commitment to their use within the hospital, and partly in the fact that the statistical tabulations yield their secrets only to those with a certain amount of skill and aptitude. Both the Commission on Professional and Hospital Activities and the Hospital Utilization Project are aware of this problem and have instituted many educational and demonstration activities to encourage the appropriate use of their products. The Commission on Professional and Hospital Activities holds about 40 one- or two-day educational "tutorials," "workshops," "seminars" or "institutes" each year at its headquarters in Ann Arbor. So far, over 4000 persons, including 1500 physicians, have availed themselves of these educational opportunities.[27a]

The medical records librarian in each hospital may prove to be a key element in the appropriate use of statistical display and analysis systems. We have already referred to her role in the preparation of record abstracts that feed information into these systems. Much more important could be her role in preparing and presenting analyses of patterns of care in a manner that can be readily used by the administrator and the medical staff in their deliberations. It has been proposed that an appropriately trained medical records librarian or other person should be appointed as a data retrieval and analysis specialist, in a staff position, in each large hospital (Slee in Reference 6, page 132). As an alternative, the staff of a central agency can perform this function for a group of local hospitals, as HUP seems to do in part.[30-32]

We have already referred to the possible opposition of physicians to the introduction of a full-fledged quality review system and suggested that, under such circumstances, a stepwise introduction might be prudent and appropriate. Fitzpatrick has proposed a similar progression, in collaboration with Blue Cross, governed by the availability of resources and the readiness of the providers of care to act. The steps he proposes are: (1) improvement of the content and accuracy of the health insurance claim form and the statistical analysis and reporting of claims information; (2) a system of statistical display and analysis based on case abstracts of all hospital discharges, for example PAS or HUP; (3) case review for suspected cases of improper utilization in Blue Cross cases only; (4) intrahospital case review for all cases irrespective of method of financing.[21]

A final set of considerations in the implementation of review mechanisms relates to the manner in which the utilization review committee is to be set up, and the guidelines under which it is to operate. For information on this matter, the reader is referred to the several formulations currently available. These include the guidelines incorporated in Medicare regulations,[15] as well as those prepared by the Hospital Utilization Project of Western Pennsylvania,[118] the California Medical Association,[117] the American Medical Association,[175] and the American Hospital Association.[176] Additional references will be found in the annotated bibliography that concludes this volume.

Costs

Information concerning the costs of quality appraisal and utilization activities is fragmentary. No report of a careful study of costs has been located. The fragments of information given below may, therefore, be inaccurate and misleading.

Morehead reports that the fee paid to surveyors in the first study of hospital care received by Teamster families was $10 for each patient whose record was reviewed. Since that study was made 10 years ago, the fee would probably have to be larger now. Morehead also reports a total cost of about $60,000 for one of the Teamster studies, probably the second. Since 430 admissions were studied, the cost per admission would be about $140. This figure includes the staff, the statistician, the photocopying (at 25¢ per page), the surveyors, the IBM and the computer runs accepted (Reference 6, page 64 and Reference 39, page 11). These are 1962–1963 prices.

Shindell reports that it cost the community about $80,000 a year in addition to the contribution of Blue Cross of Western Pennsylvania to develop the Hospital Utilization Project in Pittsburgh. However, once the program became operative, its budget, spread over 35 participating hospitals, could be completely defrayed at a cost of 42¢ per abstract (Reference 25, page 53 and Reference 30a).

The Commission on Professional and Hospital Activities charges 30¢ per hospital discharge for the Professional Activity Study (PAS) and an additional 10¢ per discharge for the Medical Audit Program

(MAP). The Length of Stay Package is an extra cost option at 9¢ per discharge if the hospital already subscribes to PAS, and 6¢ per discharge if the hospital also subscribes to MAP (Reference 28, pages 2 and 13, and personal communication).

Payne has emphasized the element of physician time in the application of internal case reviews using the "criteria approach":

> The greatest deterrent to any continuous method of evaluation of medical care is cost. The cost I refer to is the cost of physicians' time. With the growing shortage of physicians it will be increasingly difficult to involve even the most conscientious and socially aware of physicians in such a time-consuming process, and I have grave doubts as to the usefulness of any process of measurement of quality of care that neglects his involvement (Reference 45, page 4).

The cost of appraisal and review mechanisms cannot be seen in isolation. It must be related to the total program budget and to the benefits that flow from the application of such methods. Rosenfeld has referred to George Baehr's expressed opinion that about one percent of operating costs would be a reasonable allocation to quality and utilization review (Reference 6, pages 103 to 104). While the cost of review may be a very small proportion of the cost of each hospital stay, it could constitute a significant proportion of the cost of each outpatient visit. According to Slee, this might place "an important economic limitation" on the application of review activities to ambulatory care (Reference 6, page 143).

As to the relationship between the investment in appraisal methods and the immediate savings or long-range benefits to be reaped, virtually nothing is known. Rosenfeld has pointed out that as appraisal methods become more sensitive, there is a corresponding increase in cost, and one must make a judgment as to how much precision in appraisal is sufficient for the purpose in mind (Reference 6, page 36).

One must conclude from this meager collection of information on costs that preoccupation with issues of policy and technique has diverted attention from a matter of central importance: the costs of different appraisal methods and the relationship between costs and benefits. These are matters that should figure high on any agenda for future research.

Effectiveness

A fundamental question is whether mechanisms for quality appraisal and use of service are effective in altering physician behavior or bringing about organizational change. If they are effective, what magnitude of change can be expected? What factors hinder or improve their effectiveness? Finally, do the benefits obtained justify the investment in money, time and effort? Unfortunately, the answers to all these questions are rather ambiguous—but more so for some questions than others. In this section, we shall first attempt to review some of the reported findings concerning the effectiveness of appraisal and review mechanisms and then present what is known about some factors that influence effectiveness.

Findings on Effectiveness. Quality appraisal and utilization review may have at least two effects. First, the behavior of physicians in the management of care may be expected to change almost immediately due to the physicians' awareness that their practice has been made visible to colleagues and to others, and that professional and administrative supervision is in force. The magnitude of this direct, immediate effect depends on the extent to which physicians are responsive to supervision with all its implications. A more gradual —but direct—effect might be expected as a result of the educational activities associated with the analysis and review of medical care patterns and of specific instances of management. The point is that a physician's practice may be below expectation partly because of deficiencies in knowledge that the review and appraisal activities would help to rectify.

Quality appraisal and utilization review activities can also have indirect effects. These occur when the result of appraisal reveals the need for changes in the organization of care itself. Such organizational changes and program modifications can bring about far-reaching changes in the quality of care, partly through altering physician behavior and partly through other means. In the following review, the findings that bear on these effects will be grouped under each of the major methods of appraisal and control. Since most studies do not deal explicitly with the ways in which these effects come about, the reader must draw his own inferences from the data.

Certification—A number of reports deal with the influence of certification programs on the use of hospital services. Probably the analysis of length of stay distributions for Blue Cross enrollees would often show some "peaking" brought about by the acceleration of discharges at the time recertification is required. Such an effect has been reported by Michigan Blue Cross, but its magnitude has not been made public.[177] Kolb and Sidel have sought and found a similar effect attributed to the certification requirements of Medicare.[178] They compared the distribution of length of stay at the Massachusetts General Hospital before and after Medicare for persons below 65 and 65 years or older. The findings are shown in Tabulation IV-3:

CERTIFICATION

Tabulation IV-3.

Length of Stay (days)	Under 65 Before Medicare (1964)	Under 65 After Medicare (1966)	65 or Older Before Medicare (1964)	65 or Older After Medicare (1966)
Less than 14	75.5%	74.4%	63.3%	58.4%
14–17	8.1	7.7	12.4	12.2
18–21	4.6	5.2	7.8	9.9
22–25	3.1	3.1	4.9	5.2
More than 25	8.7	9.6	11.6	14.3
Total	100.0	100.0	100.0	100.0

The table shows no significant change in the distribution of length of stay for those under 65. For those who are 65 years or older there are proportionately more persons in the lower and higher length of stay categories. The particularly large excess in the 18 to 21 day category is attributed to the effect of recertification procedures. The authors point out, however, that this effect might be brought about by the later-than-usual discharge of "short stay" patients, the earlier-than-usual discharge of "long stay" patients, or both. In other words, the frequency distributions suggest a significant effect, but the appropriateness of the effect can be determined only through the analysis of individual case records. The reader should also note that (1) the differences, for those 65 or older, in the two time periods are small, though statistically significant, (2) similar changes are to be seen in the younger age group even though these changes do not attain statistical significance, and (3) the study and comparison groups differ in age, and probably sex, as well as other attributes.

A number of studies have attempted to evaluate the effects of variable-interval certification on hospital use. Zalk reports on the effectiveness of two programs introduced by a private health insurance company.[179] The first program, introduced in 1963–1964, was developed for the New Jersey Teamsters Welfare Fund, apparently at the same time the broader AID program was being developed in that

Tabulation IV-4.

Year	Controlled Admissions (1)	Uncontrolled Admissions (2)	Difference (1–2)
1963	6.73	7.72	−0.99
1964	6.02	9.32	−3.30
1965	6.45	9.90	−3.45
1966	6.45	9.10	−2.65

Average Length of Stay in Days

state. The insurance company program is said to have been well received by clients, physicians and hospitals. It also appears to have been significantly effective, as shown in Tabulation IV-4.

A similar program, developed for the employees of another large company in 48 "company locations," also shows appreciable, though less dramatic, reduction in length of stay (Tabulation IV-5).

The company attributes a savings of over $900,000 in "medical benefit claims," over a four-year period (1963–1966), to the effect of this second certification program. Unfortunately, the report of the study does not make clear precisely when the programs of certification were introduced, or whether the data cited for either of the two programs include a preprogram year. Nor is it clear how the control data were generated and, specifically, whether the control and study populations are comparable. These limitations illustrate the kinds

Tabulation IV-5.

Year	Average Length of Stay in Days		
	Actual (1)	Projected (2)	Difference (1–2)
1963	7.39	7.95	−0.56
1964	7.02	7.91	−0.89
1965	7.00	7.94	−0.94
1966	7.02	7.94	−0.92
1963–1966	7.08	7.92	−0.84

of weaknesses in study design that cast doubts on too many reports on the effectiveness of review and control mechanisms. They also highlight the need for caution in accepting the conclusions of such studies even when, as in this case, they are confidently laudatory.

A fairly serious attempt has been made to gauge the effectiveness of the AID program of variable-interval certification in New Jersey. Mikelbank has reported findings on hospital use comparing the year prior to the institution of AID with the year subsequent to its institution.[6, 23, 25] The findings are as follows:

1. Average length of stay was 7.92 days per admission prior to AID and 7.70 days subsequent to AID—a reduction of 0.22 days per admission. When allowance was made for changes in the diagnostic mix that occurred during the interval, the adjusted reduction was 0.55 days per admission. Data on comparability of the admissions by age or sex were not available for the two periods. The approximately half day of reduction "is the equivalent of conserving construction of 900 hospital beds, enabling approximately 40,000 more inpatients to be treated annually and reducing their waiting time for admission, and savings of millions of dollars to the New

CERTIFICATION

Jersey public and to New Jersey Blue Cross subscribers" (Reference 23, pages 8 and 1). However, the financial impact on Blue Cross itself is difficult to specify. Mikelbank reports:

> As far as Blue Cross saving in money, we couldn't actually make any calculation because of the fact that Blue Cross pays on a per diem rate of payment, and the per diem is arrived at on the basis of expenditure divided by the number of patient days, and as patient days went down, actually the per diem went up, so that I can't report anything as far as that aspect is concerned (Reference 25, page 74).

Furthermore, it is difficult to specify "savings" when released hospital capacity is used by patients who are themselves Blue Cross subscribers. In spite of these difficulties in defining and quantifying the savings that result from the release of hospital capacity, Mikelbank reports estimated savings to Blue Cross of 3 to 6 million dollars during the first year of AID.[23a]

2. In 100 participating hospitals, the average length of stay, adjusted for changes in diagnostic mix, was reduced in 90 hospitals, unchanged in 4, and increased in 6.

3. In the 100 most frequent diagnoses, the average length of stay was reduced in 88, unchanged in one, and increased in 11.

4. In 89 diagnoses, for at least 500 cases of which the plan paid in both time periods, the percent of cases discharged within the AID length of stay allowed was increased in 80 diagnoses, unchanged in none, and decreased in 9.

Baily and Riedel undertook a more detailed analysis of the effects of AID during the same time periods described by Mikelbank.[180] A stratified random sample of 21 hospitals was drawn. The percent of cases discharged within the limits set by the AID standards of length of stay was computed for all cases and separately for each of 11 selected diagnoses. The results for all cases in the sample hospitals for each of the four quarters before and following the introduction of AID were as follows: [180a]

Tabulation IV-6.

Quarters	Percent of Cases Discharged within AID Days Allowed
Prior to AID	
1	76%
2	73
3	72
4	72
Following AID	
1	87
2	78
3	77
4	76

It is clear that there is an immediate substantial increase in the percent of cases that are discharged within AID limits. However, equally rapidly, there is a return to a level not very different from that prior to the institution of AID. A more detailed analysis by diagnosis and by hospital showed the pattern of response to be relatively consistent in all but one of the diagnoses selected for study and in most of the sample hospitals. ". . . It would appear that as familiarity with the program was acquired, physicians returned to their customary practices of inpatient care." [180]

The authors recognize certain shortcomings in their study design. These include the unavailability of direct information from utilization committees in the stratification of hospitals prior to sampling, and the absence of contemporaneous control groups to supplement the before-and-after comparisons. Riedel has commented on the difficulty of ascribing all the changes observed by Mikelbank exclusively to the institution of AID because additional factors might have changed during the period in question (Reference 25, page 81). However, the analysis of data by quarter appears to justify the attribution of the immediate effect noted to the institution of AID.

A review of the three programs described (two private industry programs and AID) raises interesting questions, assuming the data to be valid. Specifically, what explains the apparent success of the first program, the less marked success of the second, and the disappointing performance of the third in spite of the high level of physician cooperation reported by Mikelbank?[23] In preparation for the next portion of this section, in which some factors that influence effectiveness will be discussed, it may be useful to do some speculating. In the most effective of the three programs, we are told that the physician is contacted by the "fund office" on two occasions during each hospital admission. When the patient is admitted, the fund office is notified by the hospital. The physician is contacted and told what the norms are for length of stay for the kind of case under consideration. Should the length of stay exceed the norm, the physician is contacted again "to learn the medical reasons for extension." [179] In the second, distinctly less effective, program the author's account leaves a clear impression that the physician is contacted only once, when the hospital stay exceeds the norm. There is no prior priming, as it were, of the physician.[179] The AID procedures have been described.

Necessary to the success of AID are administrative support, conscientious cooperation by the managing physician, and careful verification of physician decisions by the utilization review committee in each hospital as well as by the Blue Cross plan itself. There is no information on the degree of activity of verification procedures.

CASE REVIEW

Physicians were generally cooperative in completing the certification forms that were presented to them. But in some hospitals the entire process was sidetracked by inadequate administrative support. Certification forms were presented to the physician only after the patients were discharged and only because physician certification was necessary so that the hospital could be paid by Blue Cross. The completed forms were not sent to the utilization review committee.[23a] More recently, the New Jersey Blue Cross has taken action to strengthen several aspects of the program.[181]

Case Review—A number of studies attest to the effectiveness of mechanisms based on case review. Lembcke has reported on the remarkable immediate effects of an external audit conducted in one hospital.[41] The findings are shown in Tabulation IV-7:

Tabulation IV-7.

Consecutive 13-week Periods	Operations on Uterus, Ovary and Tubes That Resulted in Castration or Sterilization		
	Number Criticized	Number Justified	Percent Criticized
Pre-audit			
1	162	66	71%
2	156	78	67
Post-audit			
3	76	62	55
4	53	69	43
5	29	63	32
6	17	87	16
7	22	61	26
8	10	73	11
9	17	62	19

There is a clear, immediate effect. During the first postaudit period of 13 weeks, the number of criticized operations was more than halved. Furthermore, the effect was progressive and sustained. The number of criticized operations during the last two periods combined was almost 12 times less than that during the two preaudit periods.

> This change occurred without drastic disciplinary measures such as suspension or dismissal from the medical staff. A joint liaison committee representing the governing board, medical staff, and administration reviewed quarterly statistical summaries of the medical audit. The identity of the various surgeons was not divulged to this group as a whole, but the president of the medical staff, assisted by the physician members of the joint liaison committee, interviewed the surgeons with poor individual records and sought their compliance. Near the end of the fourth period the criteria and standards were printed and distributed to the staff and further improvement occurred (Reference 41, page 653).

A concurrent study of surgical operations in the community at large showed that ". . . the observed reduction in criticized cases in the study hospital was real and not due to such operations merely being shifted to other hospitals." [41]

The quasi-external audits performed by the Health Insurance Plan of Greater New York are credited by Morehead with bringing about significant short– and long–range effects through influencing physician behavior and causing changes in organization: [40]

> The impact of these studies on the medical groups was felt to be considerable. Many improvements were made in the record systems, administrative policies relating to patient care, and in the organization of the various clinical departments. The position of the "chief" of each clinical department was strengthened, as more emphasis was placed on his role in the supervision and responsibility for care provided by members of his department.
>
> Of equal importance were the measures undertaken by the Central Office of the Plan as a result of the study findings. When characteristics of the family physicians were examined in relation to their performance ratings, the relationship that was the most outstanding was the number of years of approved hospital training after graduation from medical school. The standards for new family physicians were raised to require that all applicants must have had three or more years of such training before becoming eligible to join a medical group.
>
> Another characteristic that was found to be associated with those physicians having higher scores was the amount of total practice time devoted to HIP patients. This was one added source of data which helped the Central Office to develop plans to achieve a greater number of full-time physicians within each group (Reference 40, page 8).

The excerpts quoted are a vivid illustration of the important uses of quality appraisal in planning, organization and administration. The direct educational effect is less salient and not as dramatic. In spite of sustained effort, including resurvey of physicians with low scores, only one-third of all physicians with low scores were found, several years later, to have improved in performance. One-third of such physicians had left the medical group "of their own volition, and the remaining third were still a point of disagreement between the group and the headquarters office" (Reference 40, page 7).

Morehead also attributed important effects to the studies of the quality of care received by Teamster families.[38, 39]

> The impact of the Teamster studies was considerable, both for the group sponsoring the studies and for the community as a whole. For the Teamsters, a special center was established at Montefiore Hospital for providing consultation and treatment for certain specified conditions and diagnostic evaluation for all problem cases. An educational campaign was undertaken by means of newsletters and brochures for the purpose of informing the

average Teamster family of the varying characteristics of physicians and hospitals and acquainting them with the components of good medical care. In their attempts at finding solutions to the problems facing them as the responsible agents for providing types of care to the Teamster members and their families, the emphasis of the Trustees broadened to include concern with quality performance as well as with costs of care. Following the completion of the second audit, plans were initiated to offer as a choice to eligible members a type of medical practice that would guarantee the use of well-qualified specialists and a highly organized and respected teaching hospital.

Using many of the findings of these studies, as well as others performed by the University, the Commissioner of Hospitals . . . was able to establish and strengthen codes for the performance of surgery and other specialties in the proprietary hospitals under his department's jurisdiction. Subsequently, a State Hospital Code, with almost identical requirements, was adopted equally affecting all hospitals. Payment by the City for care in special disease categories in voluntary institutions was limited to those meeting special standards, particularly those related to hospital organization and physician qualifications—the two major factors associated with high quality performance in the Teamster studies (Reference 40, page 15).

As he evaluates the information supplied by Morehead, the administrator should remember two things. First, as there is, unfortunately, no information concerning the hospital care received by Teamster families subsequent to the studies described, no actual improvement in care can be proved. Second, and perhaps more important, the use of the findings of the Teamster studies as an instrument in political strategy and tactics, though legitimate, illustrates dramatically the kind of threat such studies can pose to the status quo in the medical care system.

The case review mechanisms discussed above were external in nature. The Lembcke audit and the HIP studies also involved the identification of individual physicians whose performance was questionable and discussions with them. Other studies have shown that the effectiveness of audits is not necessarily confined to those conducted by an external agency, or to those in which individual physicians are called to task, however discreetly. Verda and Platt have reported the changes in the patterns of appendectomy that seemed to occur following the institution of a tissue committee in one hospital.[182] Over a period of three years, it was possible to reduce very markedly the proportion of appendectomies in which the pathologist noted normal tissue without increasing the proportion of appendectomies that were gangrenous or ruptured. However, a change in this direction, beginning prior to the institution of the tissue committee, is noticeable, raising the question of what other influences may have been at play during the five-year period covered by the data. More convincing evidence would require (1) a more stable baseline, (2) contemporaneous controls, and (3) some way of assuring stability in the judgments of the pathologist.

Payne has reported the extent of compliance with the criteria of good care brought about by the application of the "criteria approach" to case review in one hospital in Ann Arbor. Table 6 shows

Table 6. Compliance with Criteria of Good Care before and after the Institution of the "Criteria Approach" to Case Review in One Hospital in Ann Arbor, Michigan.

Diagnosis and Criteria	Percent of Cases Reviewed in Each Category	
	1961	1963
Urinary Tract Infection		
No stain of urinary sediment	26	1
No culture of urine before therapy	40	8
No pyelograms before 48 hours	24	28
No cystoscopy	1	3
No rectal and/or pelvic examination	63	44
No tuberculin skin test or acid fast stain of urine	24	11
Undue delay in initiating antibiotics	—	4
Acute Myocardial Infarction		
Inappropriate stay	40	21
Understay	14	11
Overstay	26	10
Cholecystitis and Cholelithiasis		
Appropriate admissions	92	96
Appropriate length of stay	72	90
Preoperative overstay	12	2
Postoperative overstay	2.7	1
Postoperative understay	5.5	2

Source: Reference 6, pages 198–200 and personal communication.

the findings. The improvement noted supports the emphasis that Payne has placed on the effectiveness of an approach to appraisal that is internal, participative and educational, and that never identifies the individual physician at fault.

Helfer has recently reported the effects of a review of the performance of two pediatric interns during their two-month tour of duty on the pediatric emergency service of a teaching hospital.[133] The method of case review was based on that developed by Williamson.[132] There were three periods of observation. The first period established the baseline of performance. During the second period the interns met with a professor daily for three weeks to review the records of cases seen during the previous day. Case review was general, and did not focus on the criteria used in the evaluation

CASE REVIEW

method. After the conclusion of the second period, the evaluation study itself was very briefly discussed with each intern and the findings, up to that point, were presented to him. However, the interns were not told what criteria were used to determine appropriateness of care. Then followed a third period of data collection without the interns' knowledge. The findings are shown in Table 7.

Table 7. Frequency with Which Specified Criteria Were Met by Two Pediatric Interns Conducting a Pediatric Emergency Service, in Each of Three Study Periods, University of Colorado Medical Center, circa 1966.

Criteria	Study Periods		
	I	II	III
History			
"Essential" items of information recorded, as percent of all "essential" items expected to be recorded *	55	52	87
Helpful items of information recorded as percent of all items recorded †	94	91	89
Physical Examination			
"Essential" components of examination recorded as performed, as percent of all "essential" components expected to be performed	79	82	93
Helpful components of examination recorded as performed, as percent of all components recorded	91	90	91
Diagnosis			
Percent of cases in which diagnosis was appropriate	95	95	100
Treatment			
Percent of cases in which treatment was appropriate	79	84	90
Disposition			
Percent of cases in which disposition was appropriate	38	53	65

* Essential items were those which staff pediatricians felt should be obtained and performed and recorded in all cases.

† Helpful items were those which the chart reviewer felt would have been helpful in each particular case.

The author concludes:

It would appear from the data in this study that merely making the intern aware of what is expected of him significantly improves patient care, measured by these criteria. The ten-minute session during which the study material was presented proved to be much more effective than the fifteen hours spent by the professors in reviewing charts. It is possible that a more specific explanation of the criteria used to determine adequacy of disposition would have resulted in additional improvement (Reference 183, page 247).

This study has several weaknesses in design and execution, including the absence of contemporaneous controls (see Zimny's discussion of the paper) and a lack of specificity in the stimuli applied to the subjects in the intervals between periods of data collection. Furthermore, the reader should be cautious in generalizing from the findings of this study, since the responses of interns in training might be very different from those of more autonomous physicians in private practice.

That physicians in private practice in a community hospital can be quite unresponsive to certain mechanisms of quality appraisal is clearly illustrated in a recent study by Williamson *et al.*[184] The study was done in a 260-bed, fully accredited community hospital with a staff of generalists and specialists. Approximately 75 percent of the total staff were board-certified specialists. The purpose of the study was to institute an educational program geared to the needs of the hospital. A baseline study showed that very few abnormal findings revealed by routine laboratory examinations appeared to be followed by appropriate action, as judged by entries in the patients' charts. It was therefore decided to build an educational program around this problem, and to try to measure the effectiveness of such a program in bringing about altered physician behavior. The educational effort began with a workshop conference in which the physicians themselves analyzed the findings of the baseline survey and decided that a "serious problem requiring immediate corrective action had been identified. . . . [However,] it was then decided that improvement in performance should be the responsibility of each individual physician [and] no group action was recommended at this time." A subsequent study of physician behavior showed no important change in response to abnormal laboratory findings. Accordingly, further efforts were made to reinforce the conclusions of the original conference. "The staff was given periodic newsletter reminders of the problem, including results of the [first] follow-up study and supplementary data regarding the criteria used." A third survey showed physician behavior in following up on abnormal findings of routine laboratory examinations to be essentially unchanged. The findings are summarized in Tabulation IV-8:

CASE REVIEW

Tabulation IV-8.

| | Percent of Abnormal Laboratory Findings That Evoked Physician Response as Judged by Entries in the Record ||
Study Periods and Intervening Events	Private Practitioners	House Staff
A. **Baseline survey**	35 (11) *	None
B. **Workshop conference**	—	—
C. **Second survey**	45 (15)	None
D. Newsletter reminders and information about criteria. Hospital obtains first full complement of interns.	—	—
E. **Third survey**	47 (13)	76

* Figures in parentheses represent "minimum adequate response."

The figures in the table indicate the low likelihood that the physician will register any response at all, and the even lower likelihood that he will respond adequately. The figures also point up the very different behavior of interns as compared to private physicians in response to the same stimulus: abnormal laboratory findings. This latter observation suggests that an organizational change, such as the institution of a training program, may be a much more effective method of achieving certain medical care objectives than attempts to alter established physician behavior. However, the reader is referred to the original paper for an account of other approaches to the alteration of physician behavior.

There is additional support for the observation that, under certain circumstances, mechanisms designed to bring about higher levels of care fail to be effective. Judging by the care provided to Teamster families, the accreditation of hospitals, which requires the establishment of a variety of mechanisms designed to improve quality, appears to have only a modest effect on the quality of care in voluntary hospitals and no effect on the quality of care in proprietary hospitals in New York City (see Table 3, page 111). It is, however, not known to what extent these findings apply only in New York City and only to care provided Teamster families.

To sum up the studies that deal with the effectiveness of case reviews, it is clear that both external and internal audits can be effective in bringing about change in physician behavior. It also appears likely that under certain circumstances favorable effects do not occur. The administrator cannot act with greater assurance of success unless there is greater understanding of what these circumstances are. Does success depend on the properties of the appraisal methods themselves, of the settings into which the mechanisms are introduced, or of both? And what are the determining factors with respect to each of these?

Statistical Analysis—There is evidence that, under certain circumstances, physician behavior is influenced by statistical display and analysis of length of stay, of other elements of physician performance, and of end results. Since case reviews are often associated components of such statistical systems, the studies described below are not clearly separable from those just discussed.

Bundesen has described the effects of introducing the "alerter system" for supervising perinatal deaths in Chicago.[83] The system includes identification of hospitals with unusually high newborn death rates, and investigation by the health department, in collaboration with the hospitals involved, of the factors that contribute to such deaths. The table below sets forth first-week death rates in 10 Chicago hospitals during the year following the introduction of the "alerter system" as a percent of the first-week death rates during the previous year. The hospitals are grouped according to the magnitude of the change observed (Tabulation IV-9).

The table indicates the range in reduction in first-week deaths (from 17 percent to 90 percent) and gives an impression of the variability within this range. More detailed time relationships are shown in Table 8 based on the experience of one hospital described by Bundesen. Table 8 shows a marked reduction in infant deaths about the time the system was introduced; but there is a gradual return to somewhat higher rates towards the end of 1954. However, the rate for 1954 as a whole does stay at about half that for 1953. Nevertheless, the suspicion remains that the effect of the system might wear off with time. There may be here an analogy to the short-lived effectiveness of the AID system of certification described in a previous portion of this section.

The Commission on Professional and Hospital Activities (CPHA) has conducted a number of studies that attest to the effectiveness of their systems of analysis (PAS) and audit (MAP), at least in certain

Tabulation IV-9.

A (Least Change)	B	C	D (Most Change)
83.1%	73.3%	51.0%	10.1%
82.5	65.2	45.0	—
82.2	—	37.4	—
—	—	36.7	—

STATISTICAL ANALYSIS

Table 8. First-week Infant Death Rates in One Hospital before and after the Introduction by the Health Department of a System of Reporting, Review and Corrective Action ("Alerter System").*

Months	Rates per 1000 Live Births	
	Before Alerter System (1953)	After Alerter System (1954)
January	13.9	0
February	39.4	0
March	22.9	8.4
April	16.7	15.3
May	29.2	13.7
June	30.8	0
July	34.0	32.1
August	7.5	14.3
September	36.8	8.0
October	49.6	15.9
November	41.7	0
December	13.7	13.9

* Chicago, 1953–1954.
Source: Reference 83, Figure 8.

situations. Eisele has reported that, in one hospital, the percent of acute lower respiratory infections that had a chest X-ray was 75.4 percent eighteen months prior to the institution of PAS, and 85.6 percent during the 6 months after PAS was put into operation at the hospital.[35] The increase of 10 percentage points could have occurred by chance only once in 100 cases.

Slee has reported the results of a more ambitious experiment to measure the effectiveness of the CPHA system and to identify some of the factors related to effectiveness.[185] The findings are summarized in Table 9. The purpose of the study was to measure the reduction in the use of antibacterials in hernia patients brought about by certain appraisal activities. All hospitals received a PAS report indicating the frequent unnecessary, and possibly harmful, use of antibacterials in uncomplicated hernia cases. Hospital Groups B and C were, in addition, participants in the Medical Audit Program (MAP) and received a special report concerning the use of antibacterials in hernia cases. Hospital Group C was the only one that participated in an intensive case review study of hernia patients. The findings show the largest absolute reduction in antibacterial use in Group C, which was subjected to all three stimuli (PAS, MAP, intensive case review), and the least reduction in Group A, which was subjected only to the first stimulus (PAS). The largest decline occurred in Group C even though the initial level of misuse of antibiotics was lowest in this group. Furthermore, the reduction in Group C occurred during the second period, possibly because of the

Table 9. Use of Antibacterials in Inguinal Hernia Operations in Three Groups of Hospitals.

Measurements, Study Periods, and Intervening Events	Hospital Groups		
	A PAS Report (N=10)	B PAS Report MAP Report (N=5)	C PAS Report MAP Report Case Review (N=24)
Percent of hernia patients who receive antibacterials. Baseline period of 11 months (January 1957 through April 1958).	40.9	40.3	35.6
Percentage point reduction in percent of hernia patients who receive antibacterials during 7 months (May 1958 through October 1958) following receipt of PAS report in all three groups of hospitals and the performance of intensive case reviews in Group C (April through June 1958).	−3.1	−4.7	−9.2
Further percentage point reduction during 6 months (November 1958 through April 1959) following the receipt of MAP report in hospital groups B and C.	−2.7	−4.6	−0.5
Total percentage point reduction in percent of hernia patients who received antibacterials.	−5.8	−9.3	−9.7

Source: Reference 185, pages 15-20.

intensive case review conducted at the beginning of this period. As a result, the incremental effect of the regular MAP report and case review activity was very small in Hospital Group C. Comparison of Groups B and A suggest, however, that MAP did have an effect supplemental to that of PAS in Group B.

The findings of this study suggest that statistical analysis and associated case reviews are effective in changing physician behavior, and that the MAP activity adds an increment to PAS. The reader must remember, however, that Groups A, B and C were self-selected, and not generated by random allocation. The design is, therefore, observational rather than experimental. Furthermore, general medical opinion during this time period tended to emphasize the need to reduce the misuse of antibacterial agents. The specific stimuli studied (PAS, MAP and case reviews) coincide with a change in the general climate of medical opinion. About 10 years later, Slee

STATISTICAL ANALYSIS

emphasized a possible synergism between the sets of stimuli (specific and general) and made only the relatively modest claim that CPHA activities help to accelerate the diffusion of new standards of practice, and to bring about desirable patterns of practice sooner than might normally be expected:

> An information system shouldn't have any ability to go against the stream of what's right or wrong. But if it's successfully employed and used, then it can accelerate the rate with which people change. For example, when there was a decline coming, if you will, in the use of antibiotics prophylactically, several years ago, we were able to look at two groups in hospitals. One in which we had evidence that they were studying this problem and the use of antibiotics just dropped off rather precipitously in a period of two or three months to a level and then held. The other group of hospitals that we could observe got to the same point about a year later. So one may be able to help accelerate communication of new knowledge (Reference 6, page 134).

Before we turn our attention to the effects of utilization review activities, it might be interesting to add a delightful anecdote, recounted by Densen, concerning the effect of statistical analysis on the incidence of puerperal sepsis in a university hospital.[186] The paper in which this account occurs is recommended reading to the administrator because it demonstrates so well the uses of statistical analysis in hospital administration.

Statistical analysis made apparent that "the concepts of puerperal fever held by the obstetrics staff at the time were not very clear." A uniform definition had to be formulated. Then it became clear that there was a previously unperceived difference between ward and private patients:

> Ward patients showed a puerperal fever rate in excess of 12 per cent, low cost private patients showed the next highest rate, and private patients had the lowest rate. The rate for ward patients seemed excessive and the rates were rising. . . . Then about April, 1945, the practice of issuing monthly reports on puerperal fever was adopted and the problem was kept constantly in front of the interne staff. They, in turn, posted a list in the nurses' station on the ward of all patients delivered and whether or not they developed puerperal fever. A noticeable spirit of rivalry developed and it came to be considered almost a disgrace for an interne to have one of his patients develop puerperal fever (Reference 185, page 1425).

> It turned out that what happened was that when the internes and residents were in the labor room (they) had a chart on the wall, and they made bets with each other as to whose patient would develop puerperal fever (Reference 6, page 141).

> (As a result) the rate for 1945 was lower than for any of the three preceding years, and for the first 6 months of 1946 it has fallen to a new low and is now at the level of the rate for low cost private patients. Since there had been no changes in obstetric practice during this time except for the exercise of greater caution in handling patients as a result of the constant

awareness of the danger of puerperal infection, the drop in the rate appears to be due to the emphasis placed upon the problem (Reference 186, page 1425).

There are a few studies of the effectiveness of statistical display and analysis, and of utilization review, on hospital use and length of stay. These studies provide information about organizational changes attributed to the institution of such mechanisms, and about changes in physician behavior as demonstrated in hospital use and length of stay data.

The agencies that have a stake in the development of utilization control mechanisms (HUP, for example), and physicians involved in conducting utilization review, tend to describe a favorable experience. Sigmond has reported findings based on questionnaire surveys of hospital utilization committees, supplemented with discussions at general meetings of utilization committee chairmen and hospital administrators in the Pittsburgh area.[187]

> Experience with utilization committees during the past few years in Western Pennsylvania indicates that they have (1) increased awareness of physicians of their central role in determining utilization rates, (2) resulted in specific administrative changes designed to improve utilization practices at a number of hospitals, and (3) improved liaison between medical staffs and hospital administration with respect to medical-administrative problems.
>
> Seventy-five per cent of [utilization review] committee chairmen reported in 1960 that they believed that reduction in "excessive stays" had been achieved; 32 per cent cited reduction in "unnecessary admissions"; and 19 per cent cited reduction in use of ancillary services.
>
> The questionnaire completed at the end of 1961 asked only about length of stay. This time, 78 per cent of the chairmen reported that their committee's activity appeared to have resulted in reduction of stays. In general, committee chairmen believed that, in addition to improvement in utilization practices, the committee had such important side effects as improvements in medical staff-administrative liaison, in charting, and in understanding of utilization and Blue Cross problems. A few chairmen also cited improvement of quality of care, reduction in hospital costs, and elimination of the need for a new wing to the hospital.
>
> A number of chairmen also reported specific changes or improvements in hospital procedures resulting from utilization review activity. Most frequently cited was improvement in hospital charting. Other specific changes reported by committee chairmen included:
>
>> Development of more equitable and efficient admission and discharge procedures.
>> Installation of the program of the Professional Activities Study.
>> Better liaison between medical staff and social service department on disposition of long-stay cases.
>> Rescheduling of "dental" cases to "dead" time in the operating room.
>> Installation of a routine laboratory unit in the admission area.
>> Institution of a 24-hour discharge notice procedure, found to be applicable to 80 per cent of the cases studied.

STATISTICAL ANALYSIS

Advance in the discharge hour.
Increased emphasis on the use of outpatient diagnostic facilities for preoperative work-up.
Requiring that the final diagnosis be placed on the chart before the patient leaves the floor for discharge.
Placing a special form on the patient's chart after some specific length of stay (such as 14, 21 or 30 days) on which the attending physician is asked to explain briefly the reasons why the patient must remain in the hospital.
Increased interest of medical staff members in working with the administration on various problems and improved liaison between medical staff and administration.
Stimulated work on newly discovered problems involving hospital procedures such as weekend laboratory coverage, operating room scheduling, and delays in tissue reports.
Focused the need to avoid delay in completing consultations.
Increased cooperation with respect to discharge hour.
Stimulated discharge or transfer to appropriate facilities for long-stay cases.
Eliminated questionable emergency admissions.

Although most committee chairmen were enthusiastic about utilization review work, some were not so sure, and many cited specific problems. Most common problem mentioned was the amount of time required by already overburdened physicians serving on utilization committees, especially the time required for essentially routine work. In addition, a number of chairmen referred to resentment by the medical staff of the committee as a police body. Closely related, a number of chairmen felt that committee members were frequently hampered because of fear of antagonizing chiefs of service and colleagues.

London [188] and Shindell [30] have commented, in a similar vein, on the favorable experience in the Pittsburgh area.

By contrast to the generally favorable opinions of what might be called "management interests," the rank and file of physicians, who are on the receiving end of utilization review, may have a less than enthusiastic view of the effectiveness of such activities. Klutch [189] quotes a study by Doyle of the opinions of staff members in two California hospitals. Tabulation IV-10 shows how physicians responded to questions concerning the effectiveness of the utilization committee with regard to specified aspects of care:

Tabulation IV-10.

Utilization Committees Perceived as Effective with Respect to:	Percent of Physicians Who Said: No	Don't Know
Reasons for hospitalization	44%	20%
Length of stay	42	19
Use of diagnostic and treatment facilities	43	20
Use of alternatives to hospitalization	39	24
Quality and costs	43	27

Some studies have gone beyond opinions about the effectiveness of utilization control and attempted to obtain data concerning effects on hospital use. McClenahan has reported small reductions in the average length of stay for inguinal hernia patients in 17 Pittsburgh-area hospitals. There was a reduction ranging from 0.1 to 1.1 days per stay in 13 hospitals, no change in one hospital, and increases ranging from 0.2–1.2 days per stay in 3 hospitals.[190] Shindell quotes data on average length of stay for 20 diagnoses in 20 Pittsburgh area hospitals combined (Tabulation IV-11). The experience in 1964 is compared with that in each half of 1965. The reductions in length of stay tend to be additive over the two halves of 1965 and to be sustained.

Tabulation IV-11.

Nature of Change in Average Length of Stay	Number of Diagnostic Categories and Range of Change in Length of Stay	
	First Half of 1965	Second Half of 1965
Decreased	14 (−0.1 to −1.9)*	15 (−0.2 to −3.1)
Unchanged	1 (0)	1 (0)
Increased	4 (+0.1 to +1.4)	4 (+0.1 to +0.6)

* Range of change in days of length of stay in parentheses.

Fitzpatrick has extended the scope of observations on hospital use in the Pittsburgh area in the hope of providing some comparison groups.[191] He reasoned that since the most intense and prevalent utilization review activities were centered in the Pittsburgh area of Western Pennsylvania, the effects of such activities should be geographically localized. Evidence for such localization was sought in hospital use data for selected Blue Cross subscribers for whom there was direct or indirect information on place of residence. The data are shown in Table 10.

The utilization patterns for enrollees of a major corporation (top half of Table 10) show that there was less increase in admission rates, and an actual reduction in length of stay, in Western Pennsylvania as compared with the rest of the state. When only residents of Western Pennsylvania are considered (lower half of table), the same effect is noted to be further localized among employees of the steel industry which is known to be concentrated in the Pittsburgh area.

The Fitzpatrick study is an excellent illustration of the use of epidemiological concepts and techniques in the analysis of medical care phenomena. However, as the author points out, the findings can only be accepted as suggestive rather than definitive. The populations might not be fully comparable and there might be additional

EFFECTIVENESS FACTORS

Table 10. Absolute Changes in Specified Inpatient Hospital Utilization Data for Nonmaternity Admissions, Selected Enrollment Categories, Blue Cross of Western Pennsylvania, 1960–1964.

	Change from 1960 to 1964		
Enrollment Categories	Admissions per 1000 Enrollees	Average Length of Stay in Days	Patient Days per 1000 Enrollees
A Major Corporation			
Enrollees outside Western Pennsylvania	10.3	0.0	10.9
Enrollees in Western Pennsylvania	9.1	—3.3	6.0
All Western Pennsylvania			
Non-Steel industry	16.8	1.2	18.5
Steel industry (concentrated in Pittsburgh area)	10.6	—3.4	6.2

Source: Reference 190, Table 3.

determinant factors in the Pittsburgh area, such as a relative shortage of hospital beds, which would influence the findings.

In summary, the evidence, mainly from the Pittsburgh area, tends to verify the effectiveness of utilization review activities in reducing hospital use and bringing about more rational use of services through changes in organization. However, the evidence at hand is by no means conclusive. Nor is there much information concerning the factors that increase or reduce the effectiveness of utilization review activities.

Factors in Effectiveness. We have already described the general factors that influence the decision to initiate mechanisms for quality and utilization appraisal, the choice among available mechanisms, and the viability of such mechanisms. These same factors also influence the degree to which the mechanisms that are instituted and maintained function effectively. Donabedian has drawn attention to certain general features of the organization of medical care that, in his opinion, either promote or hinder the effective implementation of quality appraisal and control.[5] Among the features hindering effective implementation is the tradition of autonomy in private practice, and the associated reluctance of physicians to interfere in each others' practices and to be publicly critical of each other. Morehead found the unwillingness to be critical of colleagues a significant obstacle in the performance of certain judges recruited for the HIP studies.[40]

The high degree of interdependence among physicians, with its professional, social, and economic consequences, is another major obstacle to implementation. As Donabedian has pointed out, it is unrealistic to expect a physician to be highly motivated to scrutinize the work of colleagues on whom he depends for referral. Nor is it likely that a physician on an audit committee will be overly critical when he contemplates the possibility that, as committee members rotate, he himself will be under scrutiny by the colleague whom he is expected to judge. The empirical observations reported by Sigmond support these speculations. According to surveys of utilization committee activities in Western Pennsylvania, "a number of chairmen felt that committee members were frequently hampered because of fear of antagonizing chiefs of service and colleagues." [187] If, in addition, the organized hospital staff exercises little selectivity in granting staff privileges, the quality of care is likely to be little influenced by the presence of a formal review mechanism.

Certain conditions might increase the effectiveness of patient-care review. The rise of specialization, and the specialist's desire to see his particular competence recognized and institutionalized, is one such factor. Another is the presence of an effectively organized medical staff within the hospital. Although the central importance of staff organization has long been recognized by the Joint Commission on Hospital Accreditation,[107] present levels may not suffice for reasons mentioned above. Further organization of the staff and increasing identification with corporate objectives may be necessary. This is brought about to some degree by the creation of a cadre of full-time members who can form an effective link between the institution (or program) and the private practitioner. Full-time status, especially when buttressed by membership on the faculty of a teaching institution, is associated with greater sensitivity to quality in practice, considerable immunity from the reciprocal obligations of the medical marketplace, professional prestige, and administrative leverage.

A final factor of general import is the level of professional responsibility and competence represented in the administrative structure of the institution, or agency, that finances or provides medical care. Just as physicians must be organized in ways that render them more amenable to supervision of performance and quality control, organizations that finance or provide medical care must be professionalized in order to become more responsive to the imperatives of quality practice. Several mechanisms are available for use: professional advisory committees; professional health services administrators who may or may not be physicians; and full-time professional staff to perform a variety of policy-making, administrative, technical, supervisory and liaison functions.[5]

EXTERNAL AGENCY

In addition to these more general factors, examination of the findings of the various studies that have been reviewed above suggests that the following factors may be specifically involved in the effectiveness of quality and utilization appraisal.

Presence of An External Agency—A first set of factors appears to relate to the presence of an external agency involved in the review activity. The findings, described below, suggest a scalar progression from a situation most conducive to effectiveness to one that is least conducive:

Properties of External Agency:

1. With statutory authority and direct involvement in review activities.
2. With fiscal and organizational control and direct involvement in review activities.
3. With fiscal control only, but with direct involvement in review activities.
4. With statutory authority but little or no direct involvement in review activities.
5. With fiscal controls only and with little or no direct involvement.

This scale is obviously not complete, and the reader can supply intermediate steps in the progression.

Reduction of first-week deaths in Chicago through intervention by the health department shows that the first category in the scale is likely to lead to concrete accomplishment. The effectiveness of the HIP studies might be attributed to the factors represented by the second category in the scale. That fiscal control alone can also be effective is suggested by the two studies of certification reported by Zalk.[179] These programs belong in category three. The fourth category is represented by the utilization review system under the auspices of Medicare. Whether this category will be associated with effective implementation remains to be seen. The study by Kolb and Sidel has shown some small effect.[178] However, this is reported from a hospital with highly developed internal controls, and it remains to be seen whether utilization review as prescribed by Medicare will be effective in the absence of these additional internal controls. The properties that characterize category five might be represented by the AID program in New Jersey and explain the relative ineffectiveness of this program. The Blue Cross plan was run on the assumption that quality of care, including utilization review to assure quality, is basically a responsibility of the care-providing physician and hospital, and not of the third-party payor. It respected fully the desire of the physicians to determine for themselves the quality and appropriateness of care without external interference. Even the potential fiscal controls at its disposal were seldom used. Blue Cross did not challenge any cases for any medical reasons given by an attending physician even in those hospitals where copies of certification forms were not submitted to the utilization committee. Payments were not denied even where certification forms had not been filled. Under such circumstances it is surprising that the program was as effective as the records indicate.[23a]

The activities promoted by the Utilization Review Project in Pittsburgh would seem to fall into a category intermediate between three and five and, therefore, would be expected to enjoy a reasonable amount of success.

It follows from these observations that the effectiveness of an external agency in the implementation of appraisal activities depends on the nature and degree of its power and influence and the extent to which it is directly involved in the appraisal activities.

Externality or Internality of the Audit—A second set of factors relates to the externality or internality of the audit, which in turn is dependent on the presence or absence of an external agency as described above. However, an external audit may be independent of the external agency which has a particular influence on the program. When this is the case, it is not clear whether externality, *per se*, has any special advantages. The determinative factor may not be externality or internality, but the properties of the internal organization of the program itself. When these two sets of factors are considered together, we get the following categorization:

1. External audits
   a. With high levels of internal commitment and control.
   b. With low levels of internal commitment and control.
2. Internal audits
   a. With high levels of internal commitment and control.
   b. With low levels of internal commitment and control.

Within the category of external audits there are instances characterized by great success. The report by Lembcke, which has been described in some detail, is a dramatic example.[41] There are others illustrated in the study by Williamson *et al.*,[184] in which external evaluation and participation result in failure. It is clear from the account by Lembcke that the hospital he describes was characterized by a high level of commitment to quality and readiness to take collective internal action. A contrary impression is received from the Williamson study.

Almost all the studies that have been reviewed, and which fall in

AUDIT

the category of internal audit, show that such audits are effective. These include the reports by Payne, Helfer, Densen, Eisele and Slee.[44, 183, 186, 35, 185] Some success is achieved apparently irrespective of whether the mechanism used is statistical analysis alone, case review alone, or a mix of the two. The key factor appears to be the degree of internal commitment to quality and the internal mechanism that renders this commitment operational. This is suggested by the findings of Morehead *et al.* that hospital accreditation is associated with higher levels of quality in nonproprietary, but not in proprietary, hospitals.[39]

Although the internal properties of the institution, rather than the externality or internality of the audit, seem to be the important factor in effectiveness, the reader ought to remember the relationship of the factor of externality to the implementation of quality appraisal as discussed in a previous section of this report. There is also some evidence that external standards could be more stringent, thereby presenting a greater challenge to the provider of care. For example, Myers has judged that, in 24 community hospitals which he studied, the use of antibiotics was unnecessary in 74 percent of simple inguinal hernia operations. However, the internal hospital reviewer judged that only 15 percent had received antibacterials unnecessarily.[192]

A review of selected cases in five general hospitals in Nassau County, New York, using explicit criteria developed by panels of local physicians, showed that the local hospital utilization committees tended to be much more lenient than was an external auditor at the University of Michigan (Dr. B. Payne) who evaluated each record independently using the same criteria. Part of the difference observed may have been due to greater familiarity of the external auditor with the use of such criteria. The results of these comparisons are given in Tabulation IV-12 (Reference 193, Tables 1a and 1b).

Tabulation IV-12

Judgments Made By	Percent of Cases* Admission Inappropriate (N=1206)	Percent of Cases* Length of Stay Inappropriate (N=1207)
Utilization review committee in each hospital	3.4	13.4
External auditor at the University of Michigan (Dr. Payne)	4.6	30.6

*Cases in which the judgment was "not ascertained" have been omitted. Since the cases studied are not a representative sample of all hospitals in Nassau County, nor of all cases in the five sample hospitals, the values for inappropriate admissions and length of stay cannot be generalized.

Internal Organization of the Care-Providing Agency—A third set of factors relates to additional features of the internal organization of the care-providing agency. These are:

1. Top-level support,
2. The characteristics of the chairman of the utilization committee,
3. The characteristics of the administrator,
4. The relationships between administrator and medical staff.

Little information concerning the effects of these factors can be inferred from the data on effectiveness. However, Sigmond and Shindell have summarized their experience as it relates to these factors.[187, 30]

Donabedian has pointed out that the responsibility of quality appraisal must be effectively linked with the highest authorities in any program, so that information concerning behaviors in the system can lead to appropriate structural and procedural modifications in the program as a whole.[5] This condition is implied in what has already been said concerning the presence of an external agency and its involvement in the appraisal activity. It is also a feature of internal commitment and control. Sigmond reports that the utilization committee chairmen he surveyed "were unanimous in the opinion that the committee requires the unqualified support of the medical staff's executive committee and the hospital administrator. All the chairmen with well-functioning committees reported that they enjoyed the backing of an enthusiastic executive committee."[187]

Sigmond also comments on some general characteristics of the chairman of the utilization committee:

> The chairman of the committee should be a physician who enjoys the respect and confidence of the medical practitioners. A number of younger chairmen suggested that those who have been in practice for only a few years have difficulty in obtaining full cooperation of the staff. There is also general agreement that the committee functions best when the chairman is a clinician (Reference 187, page 71).

To these general properties, Shindell has added an emphasis on certain personality traits:

> It was noted that the actual activity undertaken in a specific hospital was in a great measure dependent on the utilization chairman of that hospital. This was both a strength and a weakness of the project. . . . With an enthusiastic and conscientious utilization chairman, much would be accomplished in a specific hospital. . . . If the chairman, on the other hand, was not either enthusiastic or conscientious, there might be prolonged periods of inactivity, or expenditure of effort to justify the variant experience, rather than attempts to deal with the problems evident to outsiders (Reference 30, pages 12–13).

Shindell has also emphasized the importance of the characteristics of the administrator and the nature of relationships between him and the medical staff:

> If he was the "get along at all costs" or "don't rock the boat" type, he played a limited role either in stimulating medical staff activity or effecting necessary changes. If there were poor administration-staff relationships, each group tended to blame the other for the utilization ills (Reference 30, page 13).

Expectations of Performance—A fourth set of factors might relate to knowledge of expectations of performance on the part of the medical staff. Here again, one might postulate a progression as follows:

1. Specific knowledge of expectations,
2. General knowledge of expectations,
3. No knowledge of expectations.

As we have mentioned previously, Payne ascribes a significant role to staff participation in the formulation of criteria and to the resulting knowledge of the criteria by the staff. The study by Slee suggests that the transmittal of PAS findings (and criteria) brought about a change in the use of antibacterials in participating hospitals.[185] Helfer believes that the communication of the general expectations of performance was an effective means of bringing about behavior change in pediatric interns, and suggests that the change might have been greater if the specific criteria had been divulged.[183] On the other hand, Williamson was unable to register any significant changes in spite of considerable participation by the medical staff in the analysis of data and the explicit recognition that a serious problem existed.[184]

Feedback—Knowledge of expectations is part of a more general factor of feedback to the medical staff as a group, and to individual physicians whose performance has been questioned. Whether feedback is general, particularized, or both is of course linked to the manner in which responsibility for performance is perceived and enforced in any given agency. We have already discussed the arguments for and against emphasis on patterns of care as compared with stress on individual wrongdoing. The issue now is to see how effectiveness is influenced by one or the other of these approaches, or by a combination of the two. The individualized feedback approach appears to have been effectively used in the studies by Zalk[179] and Helfer.[183] A combined approach was also effective as used in the HIP studies[40] and in the hospital audited by Lembcke.[41] The generalized approach was effective in the experience reported by Payne[45] and Shindell[30] but not in that reported by Williamson.[184]

No clear conclusion can be drawn, except perhaps to say that generalization and individualization are themselves linked to some more fundamental factors of internal organization that determine responsiveness.

Nature of Stimuli—The nature and timing of stimuli may also have some impact on effectiveness in general, and physician responsiveness in particular. Some questions have been raised about how specific the stimulus has to be in order to be effective. It is sufficient, for example, to impress on the staff of a hospital that some method of quality appraisal is in force, or must they be informed of precisely what is being done? Little is known about this. The Helfer study suggests that a generalized review of quality was not as effective as the specific discussion of the particular study in progress.[183] Most of the other studies that have reported success have proceeded on the assumption that specificity was required.

Data are also sketchy concerning the timing of stimuli and the reinforcing effect of several stimuli. The two programs reported by Zalk [179] offer some food for speculation. In the first and more effective program each physician was contacted at the time of the patient's admission and made aware of the expectations concerning length of stay. He was contacted again whenever stay exceeded expectations. In the less effective program there was only one contact, when the stay exceeded the norm which was known to the hospital but not necessarily to the physician. The study by Slee [185] suggests that successive stimuli may have an incremental effect. Morehead has reported six-monthly resurveys of HIP physicians with low levels of performance; and the impression is that this was accompanied by improvement in performance in some cases.[40] On the other hand, Williamson appears to have failed to bring about sensitization and reinforcement through the application of two successive educational stimuli. He did, however, record response to a third noneducational and nonspecific stimulus: the obscuring of the laboratory reports by adhesive tape! [184]

Common sense would indicate that the magnitude of response would depend on how much room there was for improvement; but the relationship may not be linear. Very bad performance might be associated with factors that also prevent responsiveness to appraisal. Hence, maximum response might occur in situations where performance is reasonably good, but not too near the maximum possible. The behavior of Hospital Group C in the Slee study [185] would tend to support this hypothesis. The observations by Helfer demonstrate clearly the limiting effect of initially high levels of performance on the occurrence of further improvement.[183] When the magnitude of improvement in meeting certain criteria of performance in history

SITUATIONAL FACTORS

Table 11. Percent of Cases in which Specified Criteria Were Included in the History and Physical Examinations Recorded by Two Pediatric Interns Conducting a Pediatric Emergency Service, in Two Study Periods, and Measures of the Change between the Two Periods.*

Items of Performance		Percent			
		Initial Period	Final Period	Difference	Difference as Percent of Distance between Initial Performance and 100%
Ears	(PE)†	100	100	0	—
Mouth	(PE)	100	100	0	—
Respiratory sounds	(PE)	100	100	0	—
Duration	(H)	93	98	5	71
Nodes	(PE)	86	95	9	64
Temperature	(H)	83	98	15	88
Cough	(H)	77	95	18	78
Abdomen	(PE)	76	95	19	79
Heart	(PE)	73	100	27	100
Rhinorrhea	(H)	53	90	37	79
Vomiting	(H)	50	85	35	70
Diarrhea	(H)	43	75	32	56
Ear pain	(H)	32	78	46	68
Respiratory quality	(PE)	30	63	33	47
Drug sensitivity	(H)	5	65	60	63

* University of Colorado Medical Center, circa 1966.
† PE = physical examination. H = history.
Source: Reference 183, Table 3.

and physical examination is related to the level of initial performance, one gets the picture shown in Table 11. The absolute differences in levels of performance (column 3) show clearly increasing improvement as the initial level of performance decreases. On the other hand, there is no such relationship if one uses, as an index of improvement, the ratio of the absolute difference observed to the difference between initial performance and 100 percent. This second index measures improvement attained as related to the magnitude of the room for improvement. Incidentally, the data also show the extent of heterogeneity among different items of performance to be observed in the practice of two interns.

Situational Factors—A final set of factors that influence the effectiveness of quality and utilization appraisal may be called situational. An example is the possible effect of a bed shortage on the vigor with which utilization review activities are pursued. Sigmond reports as follows:

> Hospitals with waiting lists appeared to encounter less difficulty in getting the utilization committee functioning effectively than those in which beds were readily available. As one chairman stated, "It's difficult to sell the utilization program to your own staff and administration when there are plenty of empty beds." Action to reduce the number of beds staffed for use appears to be desirable in such situations (Reference 187, page 71).

A bed shortage may, in fact, bring about a reduction in length of stay and unnecessary admissions independently of a more formal utilization review mechanism. In this country, the work of Roemer and Shain has contributed greatly to the emphasis on the relationship between hospital supply and hospital use.[194, 195] Feldstein, however, finds that in England the supply of hospital beds influences hospital admission rates much more than it does the length of stay.[196] He surmises that physicians find it easier not to admit certain cases than to alter the length of stay norms for those who are admitted. Whether this is so would require more study to demonstrate.

Conclusion. The administrator reading this section on effectiveness of quality and utilization review may be somewhat confused and disheartened by the lack of clear guidelines as to what to do in order to ensure effectiveness. This approach to the material has been deliberate. The intention is to draw the attention of the administrator to the kinds of factors that he needs to consider in attempting to bring about effective implementation, and to suggest certain directions for further study and research. In the meantime, the administrator may draw assurance from the knowledge that under proper circumstances review activities have been demonstrated to bring about significant improvement in levels of care and the appropriateness of the use of health services.

Dangers

The possible adverse effects of formal mechanisms for quality and utilization review have received little explicit recognition, and almost no systematic study. It is true, as we have indicated, that such mechanisms are often regarded with indifference, suspicion or even hostility. However, this occurs mainly because of the general resistance to organizational incursions on the freedom of physicians rather than from explicit recognition of specific dangers to the process of care itself.

The administrator must entertain seriously the possibility that formal review mechanisms may have specific adverse effects. Payne has pointed out one possible danger: the diversion of much physician time and effort into review and control activities that are ineffective and unproductive. He suggests that certain types of recertification activity are of this nature. In addition to being wasteful, they divert attention from the application of more productive and educational types of quality appraisal (Reference 6, page 202).

Another possible danger is that formal review activities, when improperly or injudiciously conducted, will nurture dogmatism, hamper the free exercise of physician judgment, bring about unnecessary conformity, and deter experimentation and change. Densen, among others, has drawn attention to this possible evil (Reference 6, page 207). Payne, on the other hand, has pointed out that it is possible for physicians to depart from the criteria for care in individual instances, but that such departures are "conscious" rather than "unconscious," "frivolous" or "erratic" (Reference 6, page 238).

It is to be emphasized that there are no studies known to show adverse effects following the application of quality and utilization controls. On the contrary, the study of the effects of the tissue committee by Verda and Platt has shown that the reduction in unnecessary appendectomies was not accompanied by an increase in those that were gangrenous or ruptured. It was possible to reduce unnecessary surgery without hampering its proper application.[182] Similarly, the study by Lembcke showed a dramatic reduction in questionable gynecological surgery without any change in the frequency of justified surgery.[41]

Although the record so far is reassuring, the administrator should guard against the possible misuse of review mechanisms. It is hoped, and expected, that the process of review would be carried out with moderation and good sense. But, as Donabedian has pointed out, such pious hopes will not suffice. One needs procedures to ensure that supervision does not stultify initiative and change. One such procedure might be explicit notice in advance, or in the patient record, of departures from standard practice and of the reasons for them. The standards of care themselves should be subject to periodic review. In addition it would be wise to make provision, at such times, for reference to standards of care in leading teaching and research centers where the process of innovation is firmly institutionalized. A system of review which includes the examination of outcomes in relation to the process of care includes its own validating information to support or deter departures from standard practice. In any case, the procedures for review should permit a full exchange of views among the parties concerned regarding departures from standard practice.[5]

Part V:

FURTHER RESEARCH AND DEVELOPMENT

A review of what is known about methods for appraising the quality of care and the appropriateness of the use of health services confirms a record of significant accomplishment. It also reveals that there remains a long way to go. Further research, both basic and applied, is urgently needed. Donabedian has summarized the more salient items on the agenda for further research.[1] This portion of Volume II will draw heavily on that summary.

The problems to be solved seem to divide themselves into two large categories: those that relate to the ability to arrive at accurate appraisal and those that relate to successful and effective implementation. Within each of these categories one might also wish to make the distinction, difficult to define precisely, between basic research and applied research, testing or development. This general classification will be used in the discussion that follows.

Donabedian believes that further progress in the ability to appraise quality beyond refinements in methodology is most likely to come from a program of basic research in the medical care process itself. This belief is based on the premise that before one can make judgments about quality, one needs to understand how patients and physicians interact and how physicians function in the process of providing care. Once the elements of process and their interrelationships are understood, one can attach value judgments to them according to their contributions to intermediate and ultimate goals.

A large segment of the medical care process consists of interpersonal interactions between recipients and providers, and among providers. These interactions need to be studied and the relationships between identifiable features of the interactions and the end results of care should be determined. Assume, for example, that authoritarianism-permissiveness is one dimension of the patient-physician relationship. An empirical study may show that physicians are in fact differentiated by this attribute. One might then ask whether authoritarianism or permissiveness should be the criterion of quality. The answer could be derived from the general values of society that may endorse one or the other as the more desirable attribute in social interactions. This form of quality judgment is perfectly valid, provided that its rationale and bases are explicit. The study of the medical care process itself may, however, offer an alternative, and more pragmatic, approach. Assume, for the time being, that compliance with the recommendations of the physician is a goal and value in the medical care system. The value of authoritarianism or permissiveness can be determined, in part, by its contribution to compliance. Compliance is itself subject to validation by the higher-order criterion of health outcomes. The true state of affairs may be found to be more complex than this hypothetical example would suggest. The criterion of quality may prove to be congruence with patient expectations, or a more complex adapation to specific clinical and social situations, rather than the establishment of authoritarianism or permissiveness as a predominant mode. One might also discover that certain goals in the medical care process are not compatible with other goals, so that one might not speak of quality in global terms but of quality in specified dimensions and for designated purposes.

A large portion of basic research in the medical care process will, of course, deal with the manner in which physicians gather clinically relevant information and arrive at diagnostic and therapeutic decisions. Considerable work, which cannot be reviewed here, has been done in this area; but a great deal more remains to be done. The significance of this kind of knowledge to the appraisal of physician performance is too obvious to require elaboration. It is sufficient to point to the work of Peterson and Barsamian,[125, 127] and of Richardson,[128] as one application to the appraisal of quality.

A basic question that has arisen frequently in this review is the degree to which performance in medical care is homogenous or heterogeneous. A corollary question is whether there is a hierarchical progression in performance so that good performance in any given element may be assumed to imply good performance in a set of elements beneath it in the scale. Such questions have been shown to be relevant to sampling, to the use of indices in place of multidimensional measurements, and to the construction of scales that purport to judge total performance. When these questions are raised with respect to individual physicians, the object of study is the extent to which physicians integrate various kinds of knowledge and skills in their behavior. When they are raised with respect to institutions and social systems, the factors are completely different. Here one is concerned with the formal and informal mechanisms for organizing, influencing and directing human effort in general, and the practice of medicine in particular. Research in all these areas is expected to contribute to greater sophistication in the measurement of quality.

The medical care process also needs basic continuing research to validate the standards which are currently used for assessing quality, and to develop new standards. This means intensive study of end results, including the identification of relevant end results, the development of methods for their measurement, and the design of observational and experimental studies to test the relationships among elements of structure, process and end results.

In addition to defects in method, most studies of quality have suffered from the adoption of too narrow a definition of quality. In general, they concern themselves with the technical management of illness and pay little attention to prevention, rehabilitation, coordination and continuity of care or handling of the patient-physician relationship. Presumably, the reason is that the technical requirements of management are more widely recognized and better standardized. Therefore, more complete conceptual and empirical exploration of the definition of quality is needed. One important dimension that has received little attention is economic efficiency and optimum allocation of a limited resource to a specified population group, or perhaps to the management of a single person. Studies of quality should explore the implications of applying standards of "the best" care without attention to the problem of priorities. In doing so, they will have to develop methods for assessing the optimality, and hence the quality, of different strategies of allocation. There is also need for empirical studies of the prevailing dimensions and values that determine the definition of quality in relevant population groups. Little is known, for example, about how physicians define quality, or about the relationship between the physician's practice and his own definition of quality. This is an area of research significant to medical education as well as to quality appraisal. Prevalent opinions of what constitutes appropriate practice should be determined for the profession at large, and for segments of it, and compared with the opinions of leadership groups. Since the degree of consensus is likely to differ for various aspects of care, this needs to be taken into consideration. Special attention should be given to length of stay standards. The factors that determine variability within segments of the profession, and lack of congruence among segments, would need to be elucidated.

The reader may have already noticed the discussion in this section gradually approach the more operational concerns of quality appraisal. It is not possible to draw the line sharply between basic and applied research. However, in subsequent paragraphs the emphasis will be increasingly on research that focuses more directly on methods of appraisal.

One might begin a catalogue of needed refinements in method by considering the nature of the information which is the basis for judgments of quality. More must be known about the effect of the observer on the practice of the person being observed, and about

FURTHER RESEARCH

the process of observation itself—its reliability and validity. Comparisons need to be made between direct observation and recorded information, both with and without supplementation by interview with the managing physician. Recording agreement or disagreement is not sufficient. More detailed study is needed of the nature of, and the reason for, discrepancy in various settings. Similarly, the use of record abstracts needs to be tested against the use of the records themselves. In addition to checking the completeness and veracity of records, the relationship between good recording and good care should be studied. Methods of streamlining recording and making the record more easily amenable to the process of assessment need to be explored. There is also a need to develop methods for recording additional kinds of information that can be used for assessing the nontechnical dimensions of care. Attempts should be made to coordinate medical, nursing and social service records in a manner that makes the information easily available for quality appraisal.

The process of evaluation itself requires much further study. A great deal of effort goes into the development of criteria and standards which are presumed to lend stability and uniformity to judgments of quality; and yet this presumed effect has not been empirically demonstrated. How far explicit standardization must go before appreciable gains in reliability are realized is not known. One must also consider whether, with increasing standardization, so much loss of the ability to account for unforeseen elements in the clinical situation occurs that one obtains reliability at the cost of validity. Assessments of the same set of records using progressively more structured standards and criteria should yield valuable information on these points. The contention that less well trained assessors using exhaustive criteria can come up with reliable and valid judgments can also be tested in this way. The final stage in this progression is, of course, mechanization or computerization of the process of appraisal. A great deal of developmental research in this area is therefore foreseen.

There is need for more study of the implications, in terms of specificity and sensitivity, of setting standards at different levels of stringency. This is especially germane to length of stay standards and the decision to recertify at designated intervals. One needs to know what the implications are in terms of effort expended and yield achieved. More efficient methods of sampling need to be developed. The process of standard-setting itself deserves study. The reasons for inability to agree on standards would be a fruitful area of research.

There is need for much work in order to arrive at normative and empirical standards of end results. As has been noted, the paucity of such standards has handicapped the greater use of end results as an evaluative tool. Recent work by Williamson *et al.* indicates both the potential for, and the difficulties in, arriving at such estimates through polling physician opinion.[197]

Considerable difference of opinion exists among experts concerning the utility of formulating comprehensive listings of normative standards for the management of a wide range of medical conditions. The classic work of Lee and Jones [8] that attempted to arrive at such a comprehensive formulation is conceded by everyone to have important conceptual and methodological implications. However, because medical practice changes so rapidly, the applicability of such standards is thought by some to be so short-lived as not to merit the effort required to formalize comprehensive standards. Others believe that it may be useful to assess periodically current standards of practice and to explore the implications that such standards have for the planning and provision of the services needed to satisfy the standards. Falk and his co-workers are currently engaged in this kind of formulation and analysis.[198-201] The result of their work should demonstrate the degree to which such periodic reassessments are useful and should, therefore, be part of the agenda for future research.

Attention has been drawn to the little that is known about reliability and bias when two or more judges are compared, and about the reliability of repeated judgments of the same items of care by the same assessor. Similarly, very little is known about the effects on reliability and validity of certain characteristics of judges—including experience, areas of special interest and personality factors. Much may be learned concerning these and related matters by making explicit the process of judging and subjecting it to careful study. This should reveal the dimensions and values used by the various judges and show how differences are resolved when two or more judges discuss their points of view. Some doubt exists about the validity of group reconciliations in which one point of view may dominate, not necessarily because it is more valid. It would be important, therefore, to study the implications of such reconciliations. By extension, it would be important to compare the validity obtained by using multiple judges independently as compared to using them in committee. The effect of masking the identity of the hospital or physician providing care should also be studied. What is proposed here is not only to demonstrate differences or similarities in overall judgments, but to attempt, by making explicit the thought processes of the judges, to determine how the differences and similarities arise, and how differences are resolved.

As already noted, most approaches to evaluation are retrospective in nature. There is need to develop methods for concurrent evaluation that permit intervention in the process of care during any given episode of illness. In general, it is important to devise means for expediting the flow of evaluative information and of decisions based on such information.

There is another large gap in current methods of appraisal. Little has been done to arrive at an integrative appraisal of various segments of care. The methods for doing so need to be developed. Furthermore, it is necessary to develop more vigorously methods for appraising the care provided by health professionals other than physicians. Finally, ways should be found to put together the various strands of care so that one obtains a total view of patient management.

The emphasis, so far, has been on the technical aspects of the process of appraisal and the need to achieve improvements in technique. These, however, may not be the most pressing needs for further research. One can make a very good argument for the position that the present level of technical sophistication is quite adequate for most administrative purposes, and that the problems requiring more urgent solution are those that relate to effective implementation. Accordingly, it is time to get away from the exclusive preoccupation with techniques and deal with the broader issues of implementation.

Quality appraisal and utilization review activities are to be viewed as complex social interactions that occur within exceedingly complex organizations. A broad area of basic research needs to be pursued in order to elucidate the manner in which medical care organizations function and how medical care is practiced within them. The dynamics of staff organization and colleague control need to be better understood. More specifically, quality and utilization review must be seen, fundamentally, as social processes rather than merely technical exercises.

A major emphasis in this research should, of course, be on those social and organizational factors that hamper and promote the effective implementation of review and control mechanisms. Since we have already speculated at some length on what these factors might be, there is no need to attempt a catalogue of the questions that might be asked. These would include the role of external agencies in the process of control, the power relationships internal to the care-providing organization, the processes by which it is possible to achieve professional legitimation and effective group action within the medical staff, and the manner in which the review function is organized and linked to the dominant power structure within the organization.

Attention should also be directed to the possible dangers of excessive control. Although this is not likely to be a serious problem in most settings, it is an interesting theoretical problem and deserves careful study. It might provide valuable insights into professional motivation and behavior.

As has been pointed out, little is known about the costs of the various methods of appraisal, and even less about the relationships between cost and benefits. Information is needed about the costs and effects of individual methods as well as mixes and combinations of methods. The incremental costs of successive elaborations in method need to be related to the incremental benefits to be obtained. All this is necessary information for intelligent choices among the various alternatives that are open to the administrator.

Part VI:

SYNTHESIS AND CONCLUSIONS

The foregoing review of the appraisal of quality and utilization has raised a large number of interesting, and sometimes unresolved, issues and problems. A thorough grasp of these issues and problems is essential for the administrator who would want to acquire expertise in this area. But one should not allow the complexity of the subject to obscure the few simple and basic requirements that the administrator needs to meet. It is the purpose of this section to focus on these essentials.

Perhaps the most fundamental requirement of all is recognition and acceptance of responsibility for the quality of care. In the absence of this foundation stone the entire structure of quality appraisal is untenable and irrelevant. It is acknowledged, of course, that many forces over which the administrator has relatively little control may hamper his ability fully to realize and carry out his responsibility for ensuring quality. Nevertheless, the burden of this volume has been that, under any given set of constraints, the maximum possible, rather than the minimum, degree of responsibility is to be assumed and exercised. This does not mean that responsibility cannot be shared or, to some degree, delegated. Nor does it mean direct administrative control or operation of all the activities of quality appraisal. A large share of such activities may, in fact, be better carried out under the auspices of others—a medical society, or the organized staff of a reputable hospital, for example. But delegation should not mean a relinquishing of administrative responsibility. Delegation is appropriate only to the extent that it represents the most effective implementation of administrative responsibility. To the extent that it does not meet this condition, it is more in the nature of a denial of responsibility.

Before responsibility can be defined and assumed, the organizational goals and objectives, and the scope and level of concern, must be clearly set forth. Here again, the scope and level of concern should be set at the most inclusive level consistent with the mission of the agency. Similarly, the definition of quality should go beyond the merely technical aspects of care to include the many dimensions that make care meaningful and acceptable to clients, to providers, and to the community at large. The emphasis on comprehensiveness in defining the scope of concern and the dimensions of quality should not, however, detract from priorities in care. Primary responsibility would appear to be for the technical quality of the care which the agency itself provides or buys.

The administrator discharges his responsibility for quality in a number of ways. To begin with, the program he administers ought to be set up in a manner that encourages and rewards good professional performance. It should also stimulate and promote informal mechanisms of professional interaction that render care visible and subject to correction through the exchange of opinions and information among colleagues. Formal mechanisms for the review of quality and use of service are only one, though essential, element in appropriate program design.

A formal mechanism of appraisal should be set up that keeps under constant review the process of care and its intermediate and ultimate end results, to the extent that the available data permit. Program structure should also be kept under constant review, especially as experience reveals defects in process or shortcomings in end results that might be open to correction through changes in organizational structure.

It is generally accepted that the primary objective of quality and utilization review should be educational and rehabilitative rather than punitive and destructive. It is also usually conceded that primary emphasis should be on pervasive patterns of care rather than on ferreting out individual wrongdoing. However, the administrator cannot avoid the responsibility for recognizing and dealing with the particular problems of individual physicians. This does not mean that the administrator may act independently or in an arbitrary fashion. It does mean that he is responsible for seeing to it that the profession exercises the requisite degree of supervision and discipline. Concern for undesirable patterns and for individual deviance should complement, rather than interfere with, each other.

There are several methods and techniques available for quality and utilization review. More important than the technical properties of the particular method selected is the will and commitment to ensure that whatever method is chosen is made to work. A rather simple and crude method, conscientiously implemented, will be more effective than a highly sophisticated method that is half-heartedly applied or totally ignored. The administrator should, therefore, give particular attention to creating the conditions that ensure support, acceptance and implementation by the providers of care. He should also see to it that the administrative and organizational implications of the patterns revealed by quality and utilization review are explored and acted upon. This usually means the institution of cyclical activity in which the following steps recur in sequence: (1) determination of patterns of care and end results, (2) taking appropriate admin-

CONCLUSIONS

istrative action to change the organization or the behavior of providers, and (3) examination of patterns of care and end results to determine if the action taken has been effective.

The methods and techniques of appraisal and review offer a variety of choices. In making these choices, the administrator should be fully aware of the particular objectives and needs of his agency and adjust his choices accordingly. Unnecessary refinements and unused data are costly. Most administrative uses do not require very high levels of accuracy and quantification. The administrator seldom needs to place a given example of care on a precise location on an extended scale of quality. The purpose, most often, is to identify aspects of performance that may be questionable and to provide for participatory solutions to the problems disclosed through professional and administrative review. The administrator should, however, pay particular attention to the question of yield, since the constant review of professional activities that reveals nothing of note is likely to deaden motivation and bring the whole apparatus of review into disrepute. This may also happen if the premature application of very demanding standards shows everyone to have fallen short.

Possibly the best strategy in the choice of methods of appraisal is to regard the several methods as interrelated links in a system of appraisal rather than as independent entities. There is, as yet, no general agreement on what constitutes an optimal system for most purposes. The following suggestions are offered mainly to demonstrate, in more concrete fashion, the notion of a system of interrelated methods of appraisal.

The first element in the appraisal system could well be the institution of a statistical display and analysis component that focuses on the appropriate use of resources. This is perhaps the least threatening of all initial steps. Furthermore, through affording a means for comparisons among institutions, and among departments or individuals within an institution, it can impress upon the medical staff and the administrator the need for exploring the causes of variability and of deviance from statistical and normative standards.

The second step is to expand the statistical component to enable the collection and evaluation of data on professional activities and such end results as can be determined within the time limits of the data-gathering instrument.

Since the interpretation and evaluation of professional activities requires the availability of agreed-upon standards, the third step in the development of the system of appraisal might be the development of internal case review using the "criteria approach." The criteria are probably best developed by the medical staff with the aid of a manual of standards such as that assembled by Payne.[47]

The statistical component and the internal case review mechanism should be linked so that one complements the other. To the extent that the statistical component collects information concerning the criteria for case review, it will be possible to process large numbers of cases and identify those in which the criteria are not met. These would be subjected to more careful case review. Furthermore, analysis of patterns of care as revealed by the statistical instrument might lead to modifications in the normative criteria that govern case review. Because there can be this kind of linkage between the internal case review and the statistical components, the institution of internal case review might precede the institution of the statistical instrument under certain circumstances. In other words, the administrator may judge that it is best to begin by instituting the internal review and by then introducing the statistical display and analysis element as a second step designed to mechanize, in part, the activities of case review.

Needless to say, the statistical element in the system has uses beyond its articulation in the internal review using explicit criteria. The statistical component broadens the scope of analysis to reveal other forms of deviance, for example in outcomes or in the values of laboratory tests. It also can reveal deviance in the patterns of care for categories for which criteria have not been developed, and can stimulate the development of such criteria.

The fourth step would, therefore, be the expansion of the internal case review activity to include all forms of deviance revealed by the statistical component.

There is a question as to whether case review should be entirely linked to the statistical element in the system or whether it should have other inputs. It would seem wise to take the second course of action and arrange for the systematic review of selected aspects of care that are judged to be important but are not sufficiently probed by the data fed routinely into the statistical instrument. This might constitute step five in the development of the appraisal system. Its implementation might reveal problems that could otherwise go undetected. The presumption that certain aspects of care are subject to greater than usual risk of being at fault would, of course, be an important consideration in selecting them for review. This is the principle of sampling "high risk" cases as described in the text of this volume.

The reader's attention is called to the fact that not all of the case reviews envisaged above would depend on preformulated explicit criteria. The case reviews in stages four and five, at least initially, would rely on the expert opinion of the reviewers who would use implicit, internalized criteria of what is good practice. However, as

CONCLUSIONS

experience accumulates, the formulation of explicit criteria would be expected to grow, and a larger component of the review activity would become routinized and mechanized.

All the steps in the review system described so far are retrospective. Methods for concurrent review, other than those based on certification, have not been developed so far. One might, however, postulate a sixth step which would depend on sufficient refinement in the statistical element to permit concurrent evaluation and intervention during the course of management if this seems indicated.

The model described contains two major elements: internal case review with and without explicit criteria, and statistical display and analysis. There is partial congruence between the two components in the sense that the criteria developed for case review are included among the data fed into the statistical element, and the examples of deviance revealed by the statistical instrument are fed into case review. The two components are also partially incongruent since each has unique additional inputs. But the processing and evaluation of these additional inputs introduces further changes in the linkages between the two components so that the area of congruence is under constant adjustment. This model is, of course, partially hypothetical. Case review and statistical review activities have developed somewhat in isolation from each other, and the intimate linkages foreseen in the model have not been fully realized as yet. It appears, however, that this would be the natural direction in which to move.

A final point to consider is the extent to which an external agency needs to conduct appraisal activities independently of those conducted internally by the care-providing agency itself. It is the contention of this volume that responsibility for quality cannot be fully delegated. Consequently, within the limits dictated by the nature and scope of its responsibility, and the constraints imposed by the real world, the central agency should undertake the following activities: First, it should institute a method for finding out whether the appraisal mechanisms promised by the providers are in actual existence and operation. Second, it should have information concerning the findings revealed by internal appraisal and the actions taken in the light of such study. Third, it should put into operation a method for replicating, on a sample basis, the activities of the appraisal mechanisms instituted by the providers. Fourth, it should operate a system which monitors selected medical care activities and outcomes in a manner that provides an indication of the state of the program as a whole. The fourth requirement would appear to be met partly by aggregating statistical data from the several providers who participate in the program, while at the same time requiring an independent system of statistical reports at the population level.

Needless to say, there would be many obstacles, technical and political, to the activities proposed for the external agency. Here again, it might be possible to move only one or two steps at a time. Step one would be the easiest to take and step three, probably, the most difficult.

A full-blown system of internal and external appraisal of quality and utilization cannot be erected overnight. There are many technical problems to overcome. The social and political obstacles are even more serious. But the forces that call for the wider institution of quality and utilization review are powerful and equally difficult to deny. In this volume we have tried to indicate the direction of movement that these forces are likely to bring about: what the first steps might be, and how these might lead to subsequent developments.

What remains for the administrator is the decision to begin.

REFERENCES

1. A. DONABEDIAN. Evaluating the quality of medical care. *Milbank Memorial Fund Quarterly* Part 2, 44 (July 1966):166–206.
2. J. A. SOLON, C. G. SHEPS, and S. S. LEE. Delineating patterns of medical care. *American Journal of Public Health* 50 (August 1960):1105–1113.
3. J. A. SOLON, C. G. SHEPS, and S. S. LEE. Patterns of medical care: a hospital's outpatients. *American Journal of Public Health* 50 (December 1960):1905–1913.
4. J. A. SOLON. Changing patterns of obtaining medical care in a public housing community: impact of a service program. *American Journal of Public Health* 57 (May 1967):772–783.
5. A. DONABEDIAN. Promoting quality through evaluating the process of patient care. *Medical Care* 6 (May–June 1968):181–202.
6. American Public Health Association, Program Area Committee on Medical Care Administration. *Workshop on Medical Care Appraisal–Operational Aspects.* New York: November 11, 1966, 241 pp. (Unpublished transcript)
7. C. B. ESSELSTYN. "Principles of Physician Remuneration." *Papers and Proceedings of the National Conference on Labor Health Services: Washington, D. C., June 16–17, 1958.* Washington, D. C.: American Labor Health Association, 1958, p. 122.
8. R. I. LEE and L. W. JONES. *The Fundamentals of Good Medical Care.* Publications of the Committee on the Costs of Medical Care, No. 22. Chicago: Chicago University Press, 1933, 302pp.
9. M. C. SHEPS. Approaches to the quality of hospital care. *Public Health Reports* 70 (September 1955):877–886.
10. M. W. KLEIN, M. F. MALONE, W. G. BENNIS, and N. H. BERKOWITZ. Problems of measuring patient care in the out patient department. *Journal of Health and Human Behavior* 2 (Summer 1961):138–144.
11. O. L. PETERSON, L. P. ANDREWS, R. S. SPAIN, and B. G. GREENBERG. An analytical study of North Carolina general practice: 1953–1954. *The Journal of Medical Education* 31, 12, Part 2 (December 1965):165pp.
12. W. J. MCNERNEY et al. *Hospital and Medical Economics—A Study of Population, Services, Costs, Methods of Payment and Controls,* Volume 2. Chicago: Hospital Research and Education Trust, 1962, 775pp.
13. L. LEWIS and R. L. COSER. The hazards in hospitalization. *Hospital Administration* 5 (Summer 1960):25–45.
14. E. M. SCHIMMEL. Hazards of hospitalization. *Annals of Internal Medicine* 60 (January 1964):100–110.
15. U. S. DEPARTMENT OF HEALTH, EDUCATION, AND WELFARE, SOCIAL SECURITY ADMINISTRATION. *Health Insurance for the Aged: Conditions of Participation for Hospitals.* Washington, D.C.: U. S. Government Printing Office, 1966, p. 39.
16. U. S. DEPARTMENT OF HEALTH, EDUCATION, AND WELFARE, SOCIAL SECURITY ADMINISTRATION. *Headquarter Highlights* No. 27 (May 25, 1966), Page 1.
17. Blue Cross Association. Utilization review and control activities in Blue Cross plans. *Blue Cross Reports* 4 (January–March 1966):1–12.
18. L. S. ROSENFELD, F. GOLDMANN, and L. A. KAPRIO. Reasons for prolonged hospital stay. *Journal of Chronic Diseases* 6 (August 1957):141–152.

19. F. VAN DYKE, V. BROWN, A. THOM, and others. *"Long Stay" Hospital Care.* New York: Columbia University, School of Public Health and Administrative Medicine, 1963, 112pp.
20. D. C. RIEDEL and T. B. FITZPATRICK. *Patterns of Patient Care, A Study of Hospital Use in Six Diagnoses.* Ann Arbor: The University of Michigan, 1964, p. 129 and Table IV-6, p. 146.
21. T. B. FITZPATRICK. Utilization review and control mechanisms: from the Blue Cross perspective. *Inquiry* 2 (September 1965):16–29.
22. HOSPITAL SERVICE PLAN OF NEW JERSEY. *Approval by Individual Diagnosis.* Newark, N. J., 1965, 32pp.
23. G. MIKELBANK. "Approval by Individual Diagnosis (AID) Program New Jersey Blue Cross." Paper prepared for the Workshop on Medical Care Appraisal–Operational Aspects (November 11 and 12, 1966). New York: American Public Health Association, Program Area Committee on Medical Care Administration. 11 pp. and appendices (Mimeographed). (Supplementary information provided through personal communication is indicated by the superscript 23a.)
24. R. FURBACHER and G. SCHECHTER. Recertification programs. *Inquiry* 2 (September 1965):59–63.
25. American Public Health Association, Program Area Committee on Medical Care Administration. *Workshop on Operational Aspects of Medical Care Appraisal* (November 12, 1966). New York: Unpublished transcript, 114pp.
26. A. DONABEDIAN and J. C. ATTWOOD. An evaluation of administrative controls in medical-care programs. *New England Journal of Medicine* 269 (August 15, 1963):347–354.
27. V. N. SLEE. "CPHA Experience in Measuring Quality." Paper prepared for the Workshop on Medical Care Appraisal—Operational Aspects (November 11 and 12, 1966). New York: American Public Health Association, Program Area Committee on Medical Care Administration, 5pp. (Mimeographed) (Supplementary information provided through personal communication is indicated by the superscript 27a.)
28. Commission on Professional and Hospital Activities. *Brochure for 1968: PAS, Professional Activity Study; MAP, Medical Audit Program. Medical Records at Work.* Ann Arbor, Michigan, 1968. 30pp.
29. Commission on Professional and Hospital Activities. Computer analysis of length of stay. *The Record* 3, 8 (November 26, 1965), 12pp.
30. S. SHINDELL. "Hospital Utilization Review—Western Pennsylvania." Paper prepared for the Workshop on Medical Care Appraisal—Operational Aspects (November 11 and 12, 1966). New York: American Public Health Association, Program Area Committee on Medical Care Administration, 18pp. (Mimeographed) (Supplementary information provided through personal communication is indicated by the superscript 30a).
31. S. SHINDELL and M. LONDON. *A Method of Hospital Utilization Review.* University of Pittsburgh Press, 1966, 64pp.
32. S. SHINDELL. Hospital utilization-review mechanisms. *Journal of the American Medical Association* 196 (April 11, 1966):144–150.
33. V. N. SLEE. "Uniform Methods of Measuring Utilization." In *Utilization Review: A Handbook for the Medical Staff* (American Medical Association, Department of Hospitals and Medical Facilities), pp. 61–63. Chicago, 1965, 116pp.
34. E. LEIGHTON and P. HEADLY. Computer analysis of length of stay. *Hospital Progress* 49 (April 1968):67–70.

REFERENCES

35. C. W. EISELE, V. N. SLEE, and R. G. HOFFMANN. Can the practice of internal medicine be evaluated? *Annals of Internal Medicine* 44 (January 1956):144–161.
36. H. B. MAKOVER. The quality of medical care: methodological survey of the medical groups associated with the Health Insurance Plan of New York. *American Journal of Public Health* 41 (July 1951):824–832.
37. E. F. DAILY and M. A. MOREHEAD. A method of evaluating and improving the quality of medical care. *American Journal of Public Health* 46 (July 1956):848–854.
38. J. EHRLICH, M. A. MOREHEAD, and R. E. TRUSSELL. *The Quantity, Quality and Costs of Medical and Hospital Care Secured by a Sample of Teamster Families in the New York Area.* New York: Columbia University, School of Public Health and Administrative Medicine, 1962, 83pp.
39. M. A. MOREHEAD, R. DONALDSON et al. *A Study of the Quality of Hospital Care Secured by A Sample of Teamster Family Members in New York City.* New York: Columbia University, School of Public Health and Administrative Medicine, 1964, 98pp.
40. M. A. MOREHEAD. "The Medical Audit as An Operational Tool." Paper prepared for the Workshop on Medical Care Appraisal—Operational Aspects (November 11 and 12, 1966). New York: American Public Health Association, Program Area Committee on Medical Care Administration. Subsequently published in *American Journal of Public Health* 57 (September 1967):1643–1656. (Supplementary information provided through personal communication is indicated by the superscript 40a.)
41. P. A. LEMBCKE. Medical auditing by scientific methods. *Journal of the American Medical Association* 162 (October 13, 1956):646–655.
42. P. A. LEMBCKE. A scientific method for medical auditing. *Hospitals* 33 (June 16):65–71; and (July 1):65–72, 1959.
43. P. A. LEMBCKE and O. G. JOHNSON. *A Medical Audit Report.* Los Angeles: University of California, School of Public Health, 1963. 291pp. (Mimeographed)
44. B. C. PAYNE. "Use of the Criteria Approach to Measurement of Effectiveness of Hospital Utilization." In *Utilization Review: A Handbook for the Medical Staff.* Chicago: American Medical Association, Department of Hospitals and Medical Facilities (pp. 83–89), 1965, 116pp.
45. B. C. PAYNE. "A Criteria Approach to Measurement of Quality of Medical Care and Effectiveness of Use of the Hospital." Paper prepared for the Workshop on Medical Care Appraisal—Operational Aspects (November 11 and 12, 1966). New York: American Public Health Association, Program Area Committee on Medical Care Administration, 5pp. (Mimeographed)
46. B. C. PAYNE. Continued evolution of a system of medical care appraisal. *Journal of the American Medical Association* 201 (August 14, 1967):536–540.
47. B. C. PAYNE, Editor. *Hospital Utilization Review Manual.* University of Michigan Medical School, Department of Postgraduate Medicine, Ann Arbor, February 1968, 117pp.
48. G. S. KILPATRICK. Observer error in medicine. *Journal of Medical Education* 38 (January 1963):38–43. (For a useful bibliography on observer error see L. J. Witts, Editor. *Medical Surveys and Clinical Trials.* London: Oxford University Press, 1959, pp. 39–44.)
49. M. SCHAEFFER. "An Appraisal of the Clinical Laboratories in New York City." Paper prepared for the Workshop on Medical Care Appraisal—

Operational Aspects (November 11 and 12, 1966). New York: American Public Health Association, Program Area Committee on Medical Care Administration. Subsequently published in modified form as follows: The clinical laboratory improvement program in New York City, I. methods of evaluation and results of performance tests. *Health Laboratory Science* 4 (April 1967):72–89.
50. J. S. BUTTERWORTH and E. H. REPPERT. Auscultatory acumen in the general medical population. *Journal of the American Medical Association* 174 (September 3, 1960):32–34.
51. L. R. EVANS and J. R. BYBEE. Evaluation of student skills in physical diagnosis. *Journal of Medical Education* 40 (February 1965):199–204.
52. Commission on Professional and Hospital Activities. *Hemoglobin.* Professional Activity Study, Report 36. Ann Arbor: August 25, 1959, 12pp.
53. Commission on Professional Hospital Activities. *Reliability of Laboratory Determinations.* Professional Activity Study, Report 37. Ann Arbor: November 10, 1959, 8pp.
54. S. SHAPIRO. "End Result Measurement of Quality of Medical Care." Paper prepared for the Workshop on Medical Care Appraisal—Operational Aspects (November 11 and 12, 1966). New York: American Public Health Association, Program Area Committee on Medical Care Administration. Subsequently published in *Milbank Memorial Quarterly* Part 1, 45 (April 1967):7–30.
55. V. APGAR. Proposal for new method of evaluation of newborn infant. *Anesthesia and Anelgesia* 32 (July–August 1953):260–267.
56. J. C. FLANAGAN. The critical incident technique. *Psychological Bulletin* 5 (July 1954):327–358.
57. P. J. SANAZARO and J. W. WILLIAMSON. End results of patient care: a provisional classification based on reports of internists. *Medical Care* 6 (March–April 1968):123–130.
58. A. DONABEDIAN. The evaluation of medical care programs. *Bulletin of the New York Academy of Medicine* 44 (February 1968):117–124.
59. H. A. SIMON. *Administrative Behavior.* New York: The Macmillan Company, 1961, pp. 62–66.
60. G. B. HUTCHINSON. Evaluation of preventive services. *Journal of Chronic Diseases* 11 (May 1960):497–508.
61. G. JAMES. "Evaluation in Public Health." In *Report of the Second National Conference on Evaluation in Public Health.* Ann Arbor: The University of Michigan, School of Public Health, 1960, pp. 7–17.
62. O. L. DENISTON, I. M. ROSENSTOCK, and V. A. GETTING. Evaluation of program effectiveness. *Public Health Reports* 83 (April 1968):323–335.
63. H. F. DORN. A classification system for morbidity concepts. *Public Health Reports* 72 (December 1957):1043–1048.
64. National Center for Health Statistics. *Health Survey Procedure: Concepts, Questionnaire Development, and Definitions in the Health Interview Survey.* PHS Pub. No. 1000–Series 1–No. 2. Washington, D. C.: Govt. Ptg. Office, May 1964, 66pp.
65. National Center for Health Statistics. *Plan and Initial Program of the National Health Examination Survey.* PHS Pub. No. 1000–Series 1–No. 4. Washington, D. C.: Govt. Ptg. Office, July 1965.
66. World Health Organization. *Measurement of Levels of Health.* Technical Report Series, No. 137. Geneva, 1957, 29pp.
67. J. J. FELDMAN. The household interview survey as a technique for the

REFERENCES

collection of morbidity data. *Journal of Chronic Diseases* 11 (May 1960): 535–557.
68. B. S. SANDERS. Have morbidity surveys been oversold? *American Journal of Public Health* 52 (October 1962):1648–1659.
69. B. S. SANDERS. Measuring community health levels. *American Journal of Public Health* 54 (July 1964):1063–1070.
70. The staff of the Benjamin Rose Hospital. Multidisciplinary studies of illness in aged persons, II: A new classification of functional states in activities of daily living. *Journal of Chronic Diseases* 9 (January 1959): 55–62.
71. The staff of the Benjamin Rose Hospital. Multidisciplinary studies of illness in aged persons, V: A new classification of socioeconomic functioning of the aged. *Journal of Chronic Diseases* 13 (May 1961):453–464.
72. S. KATZ, A. B. FORD, R. W. MOSKOWITZ, B. A. JACKSON, and M. W. JAFFE. Studies of illness in the aged: the Index of ADL, a standardized measure of biological and psychological function. *Journal of the American Medical Association* 185 (September 21, 1963):914–919.
73. C. E. RICE, D. G. BERGER, L. G. SEWALL, and P. V. LEMKAU. Measuring social restoration performance in public psychiatric hospitals. *Public Health Reports* 76 (May 1961):437–446.
74. L. LUBORSKY. Clinicians' judgments of mental health. *Archives of General Psychiatry* 7 (December 1962):407–417.
75. E. M. GRUENBERG, S. BRANDON, and R. V. KASIUS. Identifying cases of social breakdown syndrome. *Milbank Memorial Fund Quarterly* Part 2, 44 (January 1966):150–155.
76. M. ROSENBAUM, J. FRIEDLANDER, and S. M. KAPLAN. Evaluation of results of psychotherapy. *Psychosomatic Medicine* 18 (March–April 1956):113–132.
77. D. F. SULLIVAN. *Conceptual Problems in Developing an Index of Health.* PHS Pub. No. 1000–Series 2–No. 17. Washington, D. C.: National Center for Health Statistics, May 1966, 18pp.
78. H. R. KELMAN and A. WILLNER. Problems in measurement and evaluation of rehabilitation. *Archives of Physical Medicine and Rehabilitation* 43 (April 1962):172–181.
79. C. L. CHIANG. *An Index of Health: Mathematical Models.* PHS Pub. No. 1000–Series 2–No. 5. Washington, D. C.: National Center for Health Statistics, May 1965, 19 pp.
80. D. MECHANIC and M. NEWTON. Some problems in the analysis of morbidity data. *Journal of Chronic Diseases* 18 (June 1965):569–580.
81. W. MCDERMOTT, J. A. DEUSCHLE, H. FULMER, and B. LOUGHLIN. Introducing modern medicine in a Navajo community. *Science* 131 (January 22, 1960):197–205; (January 29, 1960):280–287.
82. J. D. THOMPSON, D. B. MARQUIS, R. L. WOODWARD, and R. C. YEOMANS. End-result measurements of the quality of obstetrical care in two U. S. Air Force hospitals. *Medical Care* 6 (March-April 1968):131–143.
83. H. N. BUNDESEN. Effective reduction of needless hebdomadal deaths in hospitals. *Journal of the American Medical Association* 157 (April 16, 1955):1384–1399.
84. S. G. KOHL. *Perinatal Mortality in New York City: Responsible Factors.* Cambridge: Harvard University Press, 1955, 112pp.
85. E. G. STANLEY-BROWN, J. F. EAGLE, and H. A. ZINTEL. An analysis of operative deaths in infants and children. *Surgery, Gynecology and Obstetrics* 114 (February 1962):137–142.

86. A. M. LILIENFELD. Epidemiological methods and inferences in studies of noninfectious diseases. *Public Health Reports* 72 (January 1957):51–60.
87. J. N. MORRIS. *Uses of Epidemiology* (Second Edition). Baltimore: Williams and Wilkins, 1964, 135pp.
88. B. MACMAHON, T. F. PUGH, and J. IPSEN. *Epidemiologic Methods*. Boston: Little, Brown and Company, 1960, 302pp.
89. S. SHAPIRO, L. WEINER, and P. M. DENSEN. Comparison of prematurity and perinatal mortality in a general population and in the population of a prepaid group practice medical care plan. *American Journal of Public Health* 48 (February 1958):170–187.
90. S. SHAPIRO, H. JACOBZINER, P. M. DENSEN, and L. WEINER. Further observations on prematurity and perinatal mortality in a general population and in the population of a prepaid group practice medical care plan. *American Journal of Public Health* 50 (September 1960):1304–1317.
91. L. LIPWORTH, J. A. H. LEE, and J. N. MORRIS. Case fatality in teaching and nonteaching hospitals, 1956–1959. *Medical Care* 1 (April–June 1963): 71–76.
92. S. SHAPIRO, J. J. WILLIAMS, A. S. YERBY, P. M. DENSEN, and H. ROSNER. Patterns of medical use by the indigent aged under two systems of medical care. *American Journal of Public Health* 57 (May 1967):784–790.
93. J. N. BAKST and E. F. MARRA. Experience with home care for cardiac patients. *American Journal of Public Health* 45 (April 1955):444–450.
94. S. KATZ, P. J. VIGNOS, R. W. MOSKOWITZ, H. M. THOMPSON, K. H. SVEC, G. G. HURD, D. I. RUSBY, and F. B. WALKER. Comprehensive outpatient care in rheumatoid arthritis: a controlled study. *Journal of the American Medical Association* 206, 6 (Nov. 4, 1968):1249–1254.
95. C. H. GOODRICH, M. OLENDZKI, S. BUCHANAN, H. E. GREENBERG, and G. READER. The New York Hospital–Cornell Medical Center Project: an experiment in welfare medical care. *American Journal of Public Health* 53 (August 1963):1252–1259.
96. C. H. GOODRICH, M. OLENDZKI, and G. G. READER. The New York Hospital–Cornell Medical Center: a progress report on an experiment in welfare medical care. *American Journal of Public Health* 55 (January 1965):88–93.
97. J. ELINSON. "Methods of Sociomedical Research." In *Handbook of Medical Sociology* by H. E. FREEMAN, S. LEVINE, and L. G. REEDER. Englewood Cliffs: Prentice Hall, 1963, pp. 449–471.
98. D. G. HORVITZ. Methodological considerations in evaluating the effectiveness of programs and benefits. *Inquiry* 2 (September 1965):96–104.
99. R. C. LEONARD, J. K. SKIPPER, and P. J. WOOLDRIDGE. Small sample field experiments for evaluating patient care. *Health Services Research* 2 (Spring 1967):46–60.
100. L. S. ROSENFELD. Quality of medical care in hospitals. *American Journal of Public Health* 47 (July 1957):856–865.
101. K. F. CLUTE. *The General Practitioner: A Study of Medical Education and Practice in Ontario and Nova Scotia*. Toronto: University of Toronto Press, 1963, 566pp.
102. C. C. JUNGFER and J. M. LAST. Clinical performance in Australian general practice. *Medical Care* 2 (April–June 1964):71–83.
103. E. FREIDSON and B. RHEA. Processes of control in a company of equals. *Social Problems* 11 (Fall 1963):119–131.
104. H. H. KROEGER, I. ALTMAN, D. A. CLARK, A. C. JOHNSON, and C. G. SHEPS. The office practice of internists, I. The feasibility of evaluating

REFERENCES

quality of care. *Journal of the American Medical Association* 193 (August 2, 1965):371–376.
105. B. FERBER. Problems in abstracting and using data from hospital medical records. *Inquiry* 5 (March 1968):68–73.
106. M. LERNER and D. C. RIEDEL. The Teamster study and the quality of medical care. *Inquiry* 1 (January 1964):69–80.
107. Joint Commission on Accreditation of Hospitals. *Standards for Hospital Accreditation.* Chicago, 1964, 10pp.
108. B. S. GEORGOPOULOS and F. C. MANN. *The Community General Hospital.* New York: The Macmillan Company, 1962, 639pp.
109. J. C. DENTON, A. B. FORD, R. E. LISKE, and R. S. ORT. Predicting judged quality of patient care in general hospitals. *Health Services Research* 2 (Spring 1967):26–33.
110. M. C. MALONEY, R. E. TRUSSELL, and J. ELINSON. Physicians choose medical care: a sociometric approach to quality appraisal. *American Journal of Public Health* 50 (November 1960):1678–1686.
111. H. BYNDER. Doctors as patients: a study of the medical care of physicians and their families. *Medical Care* 6 (March–April 1968):157–167.
112. D. N. DOYLE. Accuracy of selected items of Blue Cross information. *Inquiry* 3 (September 1966):16–27.
113. National Association of Blue Shield Plans. *Methods of Utilization Control, Part I: A Description of a Large Blue Shield Plan's Program.* Chicago, 1963. 18pp. and appendices.
114. M. J. MORONEY. *Facts from Figures.* Baltimore: Penguin Books, 1967, pp. 141–215.
115. R. B. FETTER. *The Quality Control System.* Homewood, Illinois: Richard D. Irwin, Inc., 1967, 141pp.
116. H. WOLFE. A computerized screening device for selecting cases for utilization review. *Medical Care* 5 (January–February 1967):44–51.
117. California Medical Association. *Guidelines for Utilization Review.* San Francisco, 1965, 31pp.
118. Pennsylvania Medical Society and the Hospital Council of Western Pennsylvania, Hospital Utilization Project. *Guide to the Establishment and Functioning of a Medical Staff Utilization Committee.* Pittsburgh: Blue Cross of Western Pennsylvania, July 1965, 39pp.
119. L. A. YOUNG. Utilization review and control mechanisms: from the Blue Shield perspective. *Inquiry* 2 (September 1965):5–15.
120. Commission on Professional and Hospital Activities. Confidence limits for proportions or percentages. *The Record* 1, 10 (December 18, 1962), 13pp.
121. H. SAHAI and J. E. VENEY. The estimation of inpatient stay parameters. *Inquiry* 4 (March 1967):44–57.
122. F. F. FURSTENBERG, M. TABACK, H. GOLDBERG, and J. W. DAVIS. Prescribing as an index to quality of medical care: a study of the Baltimore City Medical Care Program. *American Journal of Public Health* 43 (October 1953):1299–1309.
123. M. I. ROEMER. Hospital utilization and the supply of physicians. *Journal of the American Medical Association* 178 (December 9, 1961):989–993.
124. P. J. JEHLIK and R. L. MCNAMARA. The relation of distance to the differential use of certain health personnel and facilities and to the extent of bed illness. *Rural Sociology* 17 (September 1952):261–265.
125. O. L. PETERSON and E. M. BARSAMIAN. "An Application of Logic to a

Study of Quality of Surgical Care." Paper read at the Fifth IBM Medical Symposium, Endicott, New York, October 7–11, 1963.
126. R. M. THORNER and Q. R. REMEIN. *Principles and Procedures in the Evaluation of Screening for Disease.* Public Health Monograph No. 67. Washington, D. C.: Government Printing Office, 1961. 24pp.
127. O. L. PETERSON, E. M. BARSAMIAN, and M. EDEN. A study of diagnostic performance: a preliminary report. *Journal of Medical Education* 41 (August 1966):797–803.
128. F. MACD. RICHARDSON. Personal communication.
129. R. R. HUNTLEY, R. STEINHAUSER, K. L. WHITE, T. F. WILLIAMS, D. A. MARTIN, and B. S. PASTERNACK. The quality of medical care: techniques and investigations in the outpatient clinic. *Journal of Chronic Diseases* 14 (December 1961):630–642.
130. C. R. RAO. "Problems of Discrimination." In *Advanced Statistical Methods in Biometric Research.* New York: John Wiley and Sons, 1952, 390pp.
131. H. J. A. RIMOLDI, J. V. HALEY, and H. FOGLIATTO. *The Test of Diagnostic Skills.* Loyola Psychometric Laboratory Publication No. 25. Chicago: Loyola University, 1962, 61pp.
132. J. W. WILLIAMSON. Assessing clinical judgment. *Journal of Medical Education* 40 (February 1965):180–187.
133. F. N. KERLINGER. "Measurement." In *Foundations of Behavioral Research.* New York: Holt, Rinehart and Winston, Inc., 1964. Part 6, pp. 411–462.
134. M. HAMILTON. Measurement in medicine. *The Lancet* 1 (May 10, 1958): 977–982.
135. F. E. BROWNING. "'The Record' in Hospital Bed Utilization." In *Utilization Review: A Handbook for the Medical Staff*, pp. 77–82. Chicago: American Medical Association, Department of Hospitals and Medical Facilities, 1965, 116pp.
136. J. G. ZIMMER. An evaluation of observer variability in a hospital bed utilization study. *Medical Care* 5 (July–August 1967):221–233.
137. H. B. MAKOVER. *The Quality of Medical Care.* New York: Health Insurance Plan of Greater New York, July 1950. (Mimeographed)
138. Health Insurance Plan of Greater New York. *Professional Standards for Medical Groups and Standards for Medical Group Centers.* New York, undated, 24pp.
139. D. MAINLAND. Calibration of the human instrument. *Notes from a Laboratory of Medical Statistics* Number 81, August 24, 1964. (Mimeographed)
140. M. J. HAGOOD and D. O. PRICE. *Statistics for Sociologists* (Rev. ed). New York: Henry Holt Co., 1952, pp. 138–143.
141. R. S. MYERS. Hospital statistics don't tell the truth. *Modern Hospital* 83 (July 1954):53–54.
142. F. GOLDMANN and E. A. GRAHAM. *The Quality of Medical Care Provided at the Labor Health Institute, St. Louis, Missouri.* St. Louis: The Labor Health Institute, 1954.
143. E. R. WEINERMAN. Appraisal of medical care programs. *American Journal of Public Health* 40 (September 1950):1129–1134.
144. M. C. PHANEUF. A nursing audit method. *Nursing Outlook* 12 (May 1964):42–45.
145. M. C. PHANEUF. Analysis of a nursing audit. *Nursing Outlook* 16 (January 1968):57–60.
146. A. CIOCCO, H. HUNT, and I. ALTMAN. Statistics on clinical services to new patients in medical groups. *Public Health Reports* 65 (January 27, 1950): 99–115.

REFERENCES

147. J. A. SOLON, J. J. FEENEY, S. H. JONES, R. D. RIGG, and C. G. SHEPS. Delineating episodes of medical care. *American Journal of Public Health* 57 (March 1967):401–408.
148. M. E. W. GOSS. Influence and authority among physicians in an outpatient clinic. *American Sociological Review* 26 (February 1961):39–50.
149. E. C. STEELE. Rehabilitation program in Ontario for occupational injuries. *Journal of the American Medical Association* 172 (September 1, 1960):163–167.
150. American College of Surgeons, Committee on Trauma, Subcommittee on Industrial Relations. Basic requisites for an adequate compensation system. *Bulletin, American College of Surgeons* 45 (May–June 1960):121, 122 and 131.
151. P. A. LEMBCKE. Evolution of the medical audit. *Journal of the American Medical Association* 199 (February 20, 1967):543–550.
152. American Medical Association, Commission on the Cost of Medical Care. *Professional Review Mechanisms: A Study of Selected Programs.* Chicago: The Association, 1963.
153. M. SHAIN and A. E. SOUTHWICK. State licensure regulations and hospital liability. *Public Health Reports* 81 (July 1966):581–584.
154. A. DONABEDIAN. "Quality Control in Medical Care Programs." Paper presented at An Institute on Medical Consultation and Administration in Vocational Rehabilitation Programs, School of Public Health, The University of Michigan, Ann Arbor, May 27–29, 1963. 42pp.
155. A. DONABEDIAN. "The Hospital Administrator and Assessment of the Quality of Medical Care." In *Applications of Studies in Health Administration,* Proceedings of the Eighth Annual Symposium on Hospital Affairs, December 1965, pp. 7–11. Graduate Program in Hospital Administration, The University of Chicago.
156. E. P. HUNT. Lags in reducing infant mortality. *Welfare in Review* 2 (April 1965):1–14.
157. P. G. STITT, E. P. HUNT, R. TAYLOR, and S. N. GOLDSTEIN. U.S. ranks eleventh in the care of infants. *Modern Hospital* 102 (January 1964): 81–83
158. A. DONABEDIAN, L. S. ROSENFELD, and E. M. SOUTHERN. Infant mortality and socioeconomic status in a metropolitan community. *Public Health Reports* 80 (December 1965):1083–1094.
159. H. C. CHASE. *International Comparisons of Perinatal and Infant Mortality: The United States and Six West European Countries.* PHS Pub. No.1000–Series 3–No. 6. Washington, D.C.: National Center for Health Statistics, March 1967, 97pp.
160. J. C. DOYLE. Unnecessary hysterectomies: study of 6248 operations in thirty-five hospitals during 1948. *Journal of the American Medical Association* 151 (January 31, 1953):360–365.
161. V. N. SLEE. Streamlining the tissue committee. *Bulletin of the American College of Surgeons* 44 (December 1959):518–521.
162. D. MUNRO. On choosing a surgeon. *New England Journal of Medicine* 258 (January 9, 1958):74–77.
163. National Opinion Research Center, University of Chicago. Report No. 73, January 1960.
164. J. F. SPARLING. Measuring medical care quality: a comparative study. *Hospitals* 36 (March 16, 1962):62ff.
165. U. S. Congress, Public Law 89–97, Section 1801.
166. Communication, Commissioner of Health, New York City, June 1, 1967.

167. State lists doctor standards for participation in Medicaid. *New York Times* 115 (October 8, 1966):1.
168. J. E. BISHOP. New York State's huge medical care plan for the indigent is plagued by many ills. *Wall Street Journal* 47 (August 8, 1967):26.
169. B. B. GRYNBAUM and E. SPEARE. Quality control in an urban amputee program. *American Journal of Public Health* 56 (August 1966):1199–1204.
170. R. E. TRUSSELL. Proprietary home standards in New York City. *American Journal of Public Health* 56 (August 1966):1261–1270.
171. State of New York, Laws of New York, Chapter 795, Section 2803, No. 2.
172. F. MacD. RICHARDSON and others. Rochester region perinatal study. *New York State Journal of Medicine* 67 (May 1, 1967):1205–1210.
173. H. WEST. Health insurance for the aged: the statistical program. *Social Security Bulletin* 30 (January 1967):3–16.
174. K. L. WHITE. Improved medical care statistics and the health services system. *Public Health Reports* 82 (October 1967):847–854.
175. American Medical Association, Committee on Insurance and Prepayment Plans. Guidelines for establishing medical society review committees. *Journal of the American Medical Association* 194 (November 29, 1965): 1021–1022.
176. American Hospital Association. Guiding principles for hospital utilization review programs. *Hospitals* 40 (March 16, 1966):75ff.
177. Michigan Hospital Service. *1963 Michigan Hospital Service Twenty-Fifth Annual Report.* Detroit: Michigan Blue Cross, 1963, 26pp.
178. J. KOLB and V. W. SIDEL. Influence of utilization review on hospital length of stay: initial experience at the Massachusetts General Hospital. *Journal of the American Medical Association* 203 (January 8, 1968):95–97.
179. M. ZALK. Insurance company's gentle persuasion has reduced utilization. *Modern Hospital* 110 (February 1968):102–104.
180. D. R. BAILEY and D. C. RIEDEL. Recertification and length of stay: the impact of New Jersey's AID program on patterns of hospital care. *Blue Cross Reports* 6, 4 (July 1968), 10pp. (Supplementary information provided through personal communication is indicated by the superscript 180a.)
181. G. MIKELBANK. Personal communication.
182. D. J. VERDA and W. R. PLATT. The tissue committee really gets results. *Modern Hospital* 91 (September 1958):74–75.
183. R. E. HELFER. Estimating the quality of patient care in a pediatric emergency room. *Journal of Medical Education* 42 (March 1967):244–248.
184. J. W. WILLIAMSON, M. ALEXANDER, and G. E. MILLER. Continuing education and patient care research. *Journal of the American Medical Association* 201 (September 18, 1967):938–942.
185. V. N. SLEE. "The Internal Medical Audit." Paper presented at the Annual Meeting of the American Public Health Association, October 20, 1959. 20pp. and appendix. (Mimeographed)
186. P. M. DENSEN. Administrative and research uses of routine analyses of hospital statistics. *American Journal of Public Health* 37 (November 1947):1421–1429.
187. R. M. SIGMOND. What utilization committees taught us. *Modern Hospital* 100 (February 1963):67–71.
188. M. LONDON. Medical staff utilization committees. *Inquiry* 2 (September 1965):77–84.
189. M. KLUTCH. Medical society review committees. *Inquiry* 2 (September 1965):70–76.

REFERENCES

190. E. McCLENEHAN. Hospital utilization reviews. *Journal of the American Medical Association* 196 (June 13, 1966):181–186.
191. T. B. FITZPATRICK. How effective are utilization committees? *Hospitals* 40 (September 1, 1966):45–50.
192. R. S. MYERS. The misuse of antibacterials in inguinal herniorrhaphy. *Surgery, Gynecology and Obstetrics* 108 (June 1959):721–725.
193. Nassau County Medical Society, Voluntary Insurance Committee. *Pilot Study of Hospital Use in Nassau County.* Garden City, N.Y.: November 1963, 76pp.
194. M. SHAIN and M. I. ROEMER. Hospital costs relate to the supply of beds. *Modern Hospital* 92 (April 1959):71–73.
195. M. I. ROEMER. Bed supply and hospital utilization: a natural experiment. *Hospitals* 35 (November 1, 1961):36–42.
196. M. S. FELDSTEIN. Effects of differences in hospital bed scarcity in types of use. *British Medical Journal* 2 (August 29, 1964):561–564.
197. J. W. WILLIAMSON, M. ALEXANDER, and G. E. MILLER. Priorities in patient-care research and continuing medical education. *Journal of The American Medical Association* 204 (April 22, 1968):303–308.
198. I. S. FALK, H. K. SCHONFELD, B. R. HARRIS, S. J. LANDAU, and S. S. MILLES. The development of standards for the audit and planning of medical care. 1. Concepts, research design and the content of primary physician's care. *American Journal of Public Health* 57 (July 1967):1118–1136.
199. H. K. SCHONFELD, I. S. FALK, H. R. SLEEPER, and W. D. JONSTON. The content of good dental care: methodology in a formulation for clinical standards and audits, and preliminary findings. *American Journal of Public Health* 57 (July 1967):1137–1146.
200. H. K. SCHONFELD, I. S. FALK, P. H. LAVIETES, S. S. MILLES, and S. J. LANDAU. The development of standards for audit and planning of medical care: pathways among primary physicians and specialists for diagnosis and treatment. *Medical Care* 6 (March–April, 1968):101–114.
201. H. K. SCHONFELD, I. S. FALK, P. H. LAVIETES, J. LANWIRTH, and L. S. KRASSNER. The development of standards for the audit and planning of medical care. Good pediatric care—program content and method of estimating needed personnel. *American Journal of Public Health* 58 (November 1968):2097–2110.

METHODOLOGY IN EVALUATING THE QUALITY OF MEDICAL CARE:

An Annotated Selected Bibliography 1962–1968

Prepared by
Alice J. Anderson

Table of Contents

A. Description and Evaluation of Methods of Appraisal 179
  1. General 179
  2. Certification 181
  3. Utilization Review 181
  4. Appraisal of Elements of Structure 184
  5. Appraisal of the Process of Care 185
  6. Appraisal of End Results 185
  7. Research Strategy and Design 186

B. Research Studies and Applications: Methods and Findings 188
  1. Patterns of Utilization 188
  2. Appropriateness of Utilization 190
  3. Physician Performance and the Process of Care 194
  4. End Results and Program Effectiveness 204

C. Implementation and Effectiveness of Utilization Review 213

D. Standards 217

E. Evaluation in Nursing 219

F. Drug Therapy Audit 221

DESCRIPTION AND EVALUATION OF METHODS OF APPRAISAL

General

1. DENISTON, O. L.; I. M. ROSENSTOCK; and V. A. GETTING. Evaluation of program effectiveness. *Pub. Hlth. Reps.* 83(4):323–325, April, 1968.

    This systematic evaluative approach "is based on the assumption that all programs in public health can be viewed as consisting of a combination of resources, activities, and objectives of several kinds. We maintain that each program is characterized by one or more program 'objectives,' which represent the desired end result of program activities, and that each objective implies one or more necessary conditions termed 'sub-objectives,' which must be accomplished in order that the program objective may be accomplished. 'Activities' are performed to achieve each sub-objective and consequently the program objectives. 'Resources' are expended to support the performance of activities."

    "In evaluating the effectiveness of programs, specific measures of accomplishment of each sub-objective and the program objectives, are set up, and data on attainment of each are collected systematically, following accepted principles of research design. In addition, data are collected on the extent (to) which each activity is performed as planned and on the extent to which resources are used as planned."

    Of four categories of evaluative questions the authors say are most frequently asked, this model does not apply to adequacy or to appropriateness. Program efficiency, i.e. cost, they say, will be dealt with in another paper. The authors define in detail their terms, "program," several kinds of "objectives," "activity," "resource," and three program "assumptions." Three steps are proposed. The first, describing the program, is discussed in detail with emphasis on the importance of sub-objectives and examples of just how to go about this phase. The reader is referred to other texts for the second step, measurement. Formulas are given to illustrate procedures in the third step, determining effectiveness. Ways to arrive at net accomplishment through various kinds of controls are defined.

2. DONABEDIAN, AVEDIS. Evaluating the quality of medical care. *Milb. Mem. Fund Quart.* 44(3) Part 2:116–323, July, 1963.

    A critique of evaluation methods in general, confined to the area of medical care by physicians as opposed to administrative control or cost efficiency. It examines what has been done, the merit of same, and, in the author's opinion, what remains to be done. It discusses what to assess, sources of data, sampling and selection. It examines the nature of criteria and the qualities they must possess to be useful, and such problems in the development of measurement tools as validity, bias, reliability. In conclusion, the author suggests a need for refinement in the nature of information used and in the sphere of reliability and validity.

BIBLIOGRAPHY

He believes that thus far too narrow a definition of quality has been used, and that best results can be achieved by studying the "process" of care itself. A lengthy bibliography, annotated, is added, to which the author refers the reader for examples or documentation of the text.

3. DONABEDIAN, AVEDIS. Promoting quality through evaluating the process of patient care. *Medical Care* 6(3):181–323, May–June, 1968.

   The author presents a critique of the patient care review process and makes a plea that effective use be made of current knowledge of methods and techniques. The process is presented as twofold: a set of client behaviors and another set of provider behaviors. While necessity for consideration of interaction of the two is emphasized, the paper deals mostly with issues of professional performance. The author provides a set of specifications, designed after the Lee/Jones model, as a definition of quality. Another list of "indicators" of quality, developed from components of the medical care process, is included. The paper discusses what to review, sources of information for a review, characteristics of standards to be used, objectives to be reached (e.g., education, supervision), and some of the mechanisms of the review process (e.g., examination of records versus statistical indices, implementation professionally or administratively). Finally, several aspects of the "ecology" of the review process in relation to other quality control methods are described, including the nature of social concern, and the extent of responsibility for quality control.

4. JAMES, GEORGE. Evaluation in public health practice. *Amer. J. Pub. Hlth.* 52(7):1145–1154, July, 1962.

   A discussion of the practical application of the evaluative process to public health services, including thoughts about different levels of objectives, illustrated by a dental health program. The author gives considerable attention to assumptions necessarily made when creating a new objective—value assumptions, and validity assumptions—with presentation of a tuberculosis control program as an example of how to handle assumptions. He discusses four categories of evaluation—effort, performance, adequacy of performance, and efficiency—and concludes with merits of building evaluation into a health program.

5. SANAZARO, PAUL F. Seminar on research in patient care. *Medical Care* 4(1):43–50, January–March, 1966.

   Based on firm convictions that research in patient care is vital to the development of criteria for contemporary instruction programs in clinical medicine, the Association of American Medical Colleges sponsored a Seminar on Research in Patient Care in 1965. This paper, a summary of the conference, touches briefly on such topics as: (1) "standards of research," i.e., methods and difficulties encountered; (2) definition of patient care; (3) the necessity for integrating efforts of clinicians and behavioral scientists for effective research in this field; (4) a consensus as to the desired results of patient care; (5) systematization of patient care evaluation through medical audits, tissue committees; (6) the utilization and patterns of medical care; and (7) the component elements of the medical care process.

Certification

6. FURBACHER, RAYMOND; and GERALD SCHECHTER. Recertification programs. *Inquiry* 2(2):59–63, September, 1965.

   A description of the New Jersey Hospital Utilization Project, including rationale for design and difficulties encountered in implementation. Blue Cross–Blue Shield in 1963 reduced the initial approval days from 28 to 14. New Jersey Medical Society and the Hospital Association with Blue Cross–Blue Shield formed a Committee to explore all facets of utilization. Efforts to provide hospitals with as much factual data as possible led to a 3-phase program. Phase I—compilation of background data. Phase II—comparison of length-of-stay for all minor, within major, diagnoses of each hospital against the composite picture. From 315,000 claim cases in 1963, 294,000, representing 308 diagnoses, were used for study after deleting those diagnoses with less than 100 cases for all hospitals. Average length of stay and standard deviation were calculated for each minor diagnosis; for those hospitals with no less than 10 cases per diagnosis, individual performance was shown. Phases I and II were then combined. Phase III—a listing by individual case, identifying physician involved. As of writing, an attempt is being made to arrive at a permissible maximum length of stay per diagnosis from a composite of recommendations from presidents of each medical staff. A created Department of Hospital Utilization is analyzing data and preparing studies to generate interest and understanding by utilization committees (see entry 7).

7. HOSPITAL SERVICE PLAN OF NEW JERSEY. *Approval by Individual Diagnosis.* Newark [The Plan], 1965.

   Blue Cross of New Jersey, along with Blue Shield, the Medical Society of New Jersey, and New Jersey Hospital Association, created a plan whereby a maximum number of days for each diagnosis is approved initially for Blue Cross benefits, with additional days paid for only through a physician's statement requesting continued hospitalization. A specified form for such request is filled in initially by hospital personnel, requiring a minimum of writing by the physician when additional days are seen to be needed. The manual contains a 3-digit code listing of diagnoses (cross-referenced to standard nomenclature) and the maximum days approved for both medical and surgical treatment of each. The manual also describes background analysis of data from all New Jersey hospitals which provided the rationale for the AID program (see entry 6).

Utilization Review

8. BLUE CROSS ASSOCIATION. Utilization review and control activities in Blue Cross plans. *Blue Cross Reports* 4(1), January–March, 1966.

   A description of the varied claims review committees, processes, and goals in Blue Cross Plans throughout the country, including activities of hospital utilization committees in Plans where these committees are more active. Such mechanisms as recertification, areawide planning, and educational programs are discussed.

BIBLIOGRAPHY

9. DAME, LAWRENCE R. Hospital profiles. *J. Amer. Med. Assoc.* 196(12): 1068–1071, June 20, 1966.

   This technique for hospital profiles was devised by Massachusetts Blue Cross. The actual profiles are based on the Blue Cross "population," and derived from computed actual bed use by Blue Cross members served by 136 participating institutions in the state (over 1,000,000 individual cases). The profiles present the way a hospital's utilization record appears when compared to the majority of hospitals. Profiles do three basic things: permit "comparisons"; establish "normality"; and permit "selection" of the unusual cases. Three common bases of measurement permit comparisons among facilities: (1) admission rate per 1,000 members; (2) length of stay by diagnosis; and (3) frequency of admission by diagnosis. A tolerance or "usual" range is defined as the "normal range of variations from the standard to be expected for two-thirds of all hospitals (for 17 diagnostic categories)." Standards are set on various bases, e.g., a statewide one or among only a certain group of institutions, and in relation to each of the three utilization measurements mentioned. A facility can ascertain whether a case frequency or length of stay places it outside the limits of "normality" of utilization for any specific disease category. The finished profiles show the position of the specific hospital for 17 diagnostic categories by service and contain a graphic computerized summary of unusual situations.

10. FITZPATRICK, THOMAS B. From the Blue Cross Perspective. *Inquiry* 2(2): 16–29, September, 1965.

    A critical discussion of methods of utilization review, delineating strengths and weaknesses of each, under the headings: Extended Benefits; Educational Programs; Claims Review; Certification and Recertification; Statistical Reporting as a Control Mechanism; Physician Review of Utilization—which includes discussion of the general concept, medical society review committees, and hospital committees. The number of Blue Cross Plans using each method, and specific utilization programs where pertinent, are mentioned. Administrative needs and goals are suggested. Steps to follow in a Plan's utilization program are outlined.

11. PAYNE, BEVERLY C. "Use of the Criteria Approach to Measurement of Effectiveness of Hospital Utilization." In *Utilization Review: A Handbook for the Medical Staff*. Chicago: American Medical Association, 1965, pp. 83–89.

    In order to eliminate the bias of the individual physician evaluator, which occurs in most studies of hospital use, the author proposes use of a preconceived set of criteria such as those developed in the Michigan Study of Medical and Hospital Economics by a panel of specialists in private practice and academic medicine (see entry 34). As part of the audit program at St. Joseph Mercy Hospital, Ann Arbor, criteria for five of the 18 diagnoses chosen in Michigan were refined. Work sheets were then constructed that could be completed by record-room personnel. The remaining steps of review by physicians, tabulation of work sheet data, and presentation to an appropriate body are presented. Examples of criteria lists and work sheets for three diseases are included. (Also printed in *J. Amer. Med. Assoc.* 196(12):1066–1068, June 20, 1966.)

12. PAYNE, BEVERLY C. Continued evolution of a system of medical care appraisal. *J. Amer. Med. Assoc.* 201(7):536–540, August 14, 1967.

> A description of the development of the criteria method of audit and a review of experience with implementation of this audit method by one Michigan hospital. The author presents results of a countywide and a regional project application of the criteria-by-diagnosis method, modified as required.

13. SHINDELL, SIDNEY. Hospital utilization-review mechanism. *J. Amer. Med. Assoc.* 196(2):144–150, April 11, 1966.

> Two approaches to utilization review have been developed: the case approach, and the pattern review. This paper described the method of pattern review used by the Hospital Utilization Project, developed from experience with 22 Pittsburgh area hospitals. Evolution of and motivation for the project are described. Each of the following steps in the methodology is detailed: (1) abstracting the hospital record; (2) listing of cases by automatic data-processing; (3) preparation of comparative statistics; (4) development of a hospital profile; (5) performance of individual case review; (6) identification of practices and procedures in which modification is indicated. Finally, the author relates experience with utilization review to the provisions and implications of PL 89–97. Samples of abstracts, data sheets, and graphs (profiles) are printed.

14. SHINDELL, SIDNEY; and MORRIS LONDON. *A Method of Hospital Utilization Review*. Pittsburgh: University of Pittsburgh Press, 1966, 64 pp.

> This manual is subsequent to "Guide to the Establishment and Functioning of a Medical Staff Utilization Committee,"* and meant for institutions yet to formulate a committee. It is an exposition of the method evolved by HUP in the Pittsburgh area.
>
> **Chapter I.** Contains discussion of: a sample abstract of a hospital record; sample of printout of a series of cases; sample analysis of comparative experience among hospitals; development of a hospital profile; studies of individual cases; data obtainable from individual cases; sample studies of practice and procedures.
>
> **Chapter II.** Specific instructions for abstracting the medical record, with illustrations.
>
> **Chapter III.** Description of various products which emerge from the data processing (computer printouts). Sections, with illustrations, on: the monthly diagnosis and operation listings; reading the basic printout; summary data on the basic listings; using the basic printout; the monthly discharge analysis.
>
> **Chapter IV.** Detailed steps to be followed in individual case review. Tables and work sheets included.
>
> **Chapter V.** Discussion of reviewing internal [institutional] practices using an OR study to illustrate.

15. SLEE, VERGIL. Medical Audit is best method of meeting utilization review need. *Modern Hospital* 105(6):70–72, 128, December, 1965.

> The author suggests a mechanism for review of the medical necessity for inpatient service of extended duration. The review done on specified

---
* Reprinted as Chapter VI of this manual. See entry 83.

days and called "medical necessity determination," is for on-the-spot reviews. A second mechanism, utilization evaluation, a retrospective review of admission, duration of stay, and professional services furnished, is also suggested. Both mechanisms are to be handled separately. The first mechanism requires tagging each admission, establishing a reminder for the daily review system, evaluating necessity for hospitalization, etc. The second mechanism is related to the internal medical audit though it is stated that the term *medical audit* has a more general meaning, and utilization evaluation is only part of the audit's total function. Utilization evaluation is an effort to control use of facilities and resources, while the audit is mainly a weapon against "obsolescence" of the medical audit committee.

16. SLEE, VERGIL. Information systems and measurement tools. *J. Amer. Med. Assoc.* 196(12):1063–1065, June 20, 1966.

    Slee's emphasis is on an explanation of the functioning of the Professional Activities Study (PAS) and the Medical Audit Program (MAP), systems offered by the Commission on Professional and Hospital Activities (CPHA), which he feels bridge the gap between the two unsatisfactory sources of medical care information: (1) the *original* clinical record or (2) statistical profiles. Three unique aspects of the CPHA method are enumerated: (1) "reliance on an extensive, single, standardized abstract for all kinds of cases"; (2) sophisticated automated information handling; and (3) depth of investigation possible without access to the original records. Medicare Act utilization review regulations are discussed in terms of "medical necessity determination" and "utilization evaluation." Certain other dichotomies in various aspects of utilization review are discussed, e.g., differences between a medical audit and utilization evaluation, and two problems involved in utilization studies—establishment of standards and ascertaining kind of care rendered.

17. STURGES, JOHN P. JR. The inpatient discharge statistics program. *Inquiry* 2(2):39–42, September, 1965.

    This IDS program, of Blue Cross of Northeast Ohio for the Cleveland Hospital Study, aims to provide hospitals with the mechanization for keeping statistics, and to accumulate these data for planning purposes. The author briefly describes the eight monthly reports sent to each hospital; discharge journal; financial class report; geographic origin report; discharge analysis by service; physicians' index; consulting physicians' index. Some of the problems encountered in establishing and maintaining the program are mentioned.

Appraisal of Elements of Structure

18. MEDICAL CARE STUDIES UNIT. *Development of a Hospital Service Index.* Medical Care Studies Pub. No. 2. Berkeley: California State Department of Public Health, 1965.

    Under the direction of Walter Bruce and Lester Breslow, this index was devised to "evaluate every significant factor which contributes to quality of hospital services," especially for county hospitals of California. It was compiled from factors derived from other studies, consultation with experts, and experience of the staff. From an outline of nine categories (such as preventive services, rehabilitative services, administration of care, availability), individual items requiring a "yes" or "no" answer were devised for each. Results of a pilot study using available data for the county hospitals were compared with results of subjective ratings by field representatives of the Bureau of Hospitals, and good correlation was found. A more extensive format was then adopted and the information was to be collected by direct visits to the hospitals. A field trial of this index (provided in entirety in an appendix), consisting of 121 items, used a weighted scoring system. Further revisions into 135 items arrayed into 20 subindices produced the final index with which a direct scoring method was applied. This version is also given. Scoring results of the first field test are provided, and rationale for the weighted scores is explained.

Appraisal of the Process of Care

19. LEMBCKE, PAUL A. Evolution of the medical audit. *J. Amer. Med. Assoc.* 199(8):543–550, February 20, 1967.

   An historical review of the medical audit from the Flexner Report and the "End Result" system by Codman through "hospital standardization," accreditation, and "Reports of Professional Activities" in the Rochester region, to more current systems and efforts. An extensive list of references to key papers on the medical audit as it developed through the years is included.

20. MOREHEAD, MILDRED A. The medical audit as an operational tool. *Amer. J. Pub. Hlth.* 57(9):1643–1656, September, 1967.

   This paper is an intensive critique of major medical audit efforts as conducted by HIP and in behalf of Teamster families in New York City, the second having been considerably influenced by the HIP experience. The designs of the studies, methods and criteria used, and problems encountered in arriving at satisfactory scoring, are detailed for each. Desirable qualifications for surveyors (judges) and some policy changes resulting from the studies are also discussed. Included is a sample of the scoring card used in the HIP Studies.

Appraisal of End Results

21. SANDERS, BARKEV S. Measuring community health levels. *Amer. J. Pub. Hlth.* 54(7):1063–1070, July, 1964.

   This paper attacks the popular assumption that high morbidity connotes deficient health care, and proposes that the end product, productive man-years, be used as a measure. The author refutes the morbidity theory by citing high rating in traditional indices of health care (such as infant mortality rates, standardized death rates, preventive services) in the example of Kit Carson County Survey findings, despite the very high morbidity rates there. He also points out that the chronic conditions at the top of the list found in the Baltimore study are those still defying very effective control. In addition to disease prevalence due to prolongation of life, he suggests that there may be an increase in the number of persons with low health potential in the newborn population. Further, present volume-of-morbidity measures take no consideration of genetic differences. The author proposes the functional adequacy of an individual to fulfill a role in society as a possibly better measure of health. A life table would be constructed to determine probability of functional effectiveness as well as probable survival; productive man-years per 100,000 might then be high in a community with high age-specific morbidity rates for chronic conditions. Methods for appraising comparative adequacy of health care by communities are presented.

22. SHAPIRO, SAM. End result measurements of quality of medical care. *Milb. Mem. Fund Quart.* 45(2):7–30, April, 1967.

A review of some completed end-result studies and some others in progress, with an assessment of weaknesses, needs, and the future of such research. Examples of completed studies are taken entirely from HIP experience. For discussion of some efforts underway, the author chooses a study of: health maintenance services for a chronic-disease population (Cleveland, prepaid group); health status of newborns in an MIC program (California); personal health services under varied care settings, and one to measure outcomes of medical care as related to patient, doctor, and hospital characteristics. This paper includes a discussion of two intensive screening-program studies, each using a control group of patients.

Research Strategy and Design

23. HORVITZ, DAVID G. Methodological considerations in evaluating the effectiveness of programs and benefits. *Inquiry* 2(2):96–104, September, 1965.

This paper discusses salient features of research design and methodology, such as: retrospective and prospective studies; dependent variables and how they can be controlled; experimental error; sensitivity; factorial design; Latin square; and rotation designs. Examples of how these various methods may be applied to different kinds of utilization data are offered. In addition to recommending controlled experimentation in hospital utilization evaluation, the author advocates the participation of a number of insurance plans in a cooperative research program.

24. SUCHMAN, EDWARD A. *Evaluative Research: Principles and Practice in Public Service and Social Action Programs.* New York: Russell Sage Foundation, 1967.

This work deals with the conceptual, methodological, and administrative aspects of evaluation applied to public service and social action programs, with emphasis on evaluative research as a method for studying the effectiveness of efforts at planned social change.

"The book is divided into three main sections, representing the conceptual, the methodological, and the administrative aspects of evaluation. We begin with a brief, historical account of evaluative research and a general critique of the current status of evaluation studies, with particular emphasis upon the shortcomings of many of the evaluation guides proposed for community self-surveys of public service programs (Chapter II). This introduction is followed by a conceptual analysis of the evaluation process, including a definition of evaluative research and the place of values, objectives, and assumptions in such research (Chapter III), and concluding with an analysis of different levels of objectives and categories of evaluation (Chapter IV).

"The next three chapters deal with methodological problems in evaluative research. We begin by comparing evaluative with nonevaluative research, summarizing different approaches to evaluation, and discussing the formulation of an evaluative research problem (Chapter V). An analysis of various research designs applicable to evaluative research is presented in the following chapter, with detailed emphasis being given to the three main conditions of an evaluative research design: (1) sampling equivalent experimental and control groups, (2) isolation and control of the stimulus, and (3) definition and measurement of the criteria of effect (Chapter VI). The final chapter on methodology takes up the problems of reliability, validity, and differential results in the measurement of the effects of a program (Chapter VII).

"Administrative aspects of evaluation are discussed next; first, the place of evaluation in the administrative process as related to program planning, demonstration, and operation, including an analysis of administrative resistance and barriers to evaluation (Chapter VIII); and second, problems in the administration of evaluation studies, such as resources, role relationships, the carrying-out of an evaluation study, and the utilization (or nonutilization) of findings (Chapter IX).

"The book concludes with a brief exposition on the relationship of evaluative research to social experimentation, stressing the potential contribution which public service and social action programs can make to our knowledge of administrative science and social change (Chapter X)."

25. SUSSMAN, MARVIN B. "Use of the Longitudinal Design in Studies of Long Term Illness: Some Advantages and Limitations." In *Symposium on Research in Long-Term Care.* Proceedings. [Jewish Hospital of St. Louis], 1963, pp. 17–32.

Advantages and problems connected with longitudinal designs are analyzed. Six variables concerned with internal validity and which must be controlled are examined. Then two examples of longitudinal studies are described. In the first, effects of tuberculosis on the social and vocational activities of individuals after hospital discharge were studied. A case register of each patient was kept for five years after discharge. On a sample of 400 out of 6,000 cases, socioeconomic variables deemed important to the patient's adjustment were delineated from this register and interviews with the patient. An extension of the study to a sample of 353 newly-discharged first admissions tested data from the pilot study and that concerned with social, economic, vocational, and medical phenomena to isolate predictable characteristics. Hypotheses were formulated from indices validated in the first study of 400. Problems confounding this project are explored.

The second reported project concerned the effect of change in structure and function of a 15-clinic outpatient department of a large teaching hospital on staff and patient satisfaction with medical care. Experimental and control groups were studied before and after change. Difficulties of evaluation in a hospital setting and problems in establishing validity and control of variables are detailed. The author concludes that invalidity should not deter one from a longitudinal design but that the researcher should try to apply tighter controls and new techniques.

RESEARCH STUDIES AND APPLICATIONS: METHODS AND FINDINGS

Patterns of Utilization

26. COMMISSION ON PROFESSIONAL AND HOSPITAL ACTIVITIES. *Length of Stay in Short Term General Hospitals: (1963–1964)*. New York, McGraw-Hill, 1966, 216 pp.

    This is a compilation of the PAS computed, stratified statistics described in entry 27. The book consists of tables describing the length-of-stay distribution for 3,660 strata.

27. LEIGHTON, ERIC; and PETER HEADLEY. Computer analysis of length of stay. *Hosp. Prog.* 49(4):67–70, April, 1968.

    A computer analysis of PAS data was designed to diminish the effects of patient characteristics, hence allow physicians to see effects of their own decision-making. Data were stratified according to: final diagnosis, patient age, whether surgery was performed, and whether there were secondary diagnoses. Statistics were calculated for: length-of-stay distribution, average stay, variance, and various percentiles; these constituted the master table. The program was then devised to match a patient with the proper stratum in the master table. The program also includes a test for significance in the difference. Illustrations are given of how the technique can be used to compare physicians with each other and one hospital with another.

28. MCCORKLE, LOIS P. Utilization of facilities of a university hospital: length of inpatient stay in various departments. *Hlth. Serv. Res.* 1(1):91–114, Summer, 1966.

    (Journal Summary) The lengths of hospital stay among adult inpatients discharged during 1962 from the medical and surgical specialty departments of a large urban university-affiliated general hospital [Cleveland] have been examined. Data are shown comparing the durations of hospitalization of patients who had a private physician directly responsible for their hospital care (private patients) and of those who did not (staff patients). The relation between the lengths of stay of private patients and those of staff patients varied considerably from one hospital department to another. On the medical services, staff patients had longer hospital stays than did private patients, a discrepancy that could not be accounted for by differences between the two groups in age, race, sex, or source of payment for hospitalization and it is being studied further. A major cause of the apparent difference in lengths of hospitalization between private and staff surgical patients proved to be inconsistencies in the criteria used to define the terms "hospital admission" and "inpatient" among various patient groups. Some of the possible effects of variations in the definition of these terms and the terms "medical patients" and "surgical patients" in hospital-use studies are discussed.

29. MASSACHUSETTS BLUE CROSS, INC., OFFICE OF RESEARCH. *1965 Patient Profiles—Average Stay, 44 Most Frequent Diagnoses.* Boston: The Office, October, 1967. 48 pp.

"In September 1967, the Massachusetts Blue Cross Research Department published a study which recorded the average stay and other information about the most frequent diagnoses by various categories of service, sex and age. This was based on 1965 Blue Cross admissions processed in 132 Massachusetts Blue Cross participating short-term general hospitals. The September study displayed a total of 86 diagnoses since diagnoses varied from one category to another with respect to frequency. "For this presentation, the results of the statewide analysis are compared with corresponding results developed from study of the Hospital Groups comprising the statewide population. This analysis was conducted with respect to the average stay experienced for the twenty most frequent medical diagnoses, the twenty most frequent surgical diagnoses and the four most frequent obstetrical diagnoses.

"The diagnoses included herein are judged the most frequent on the basis of statewide case frequency, all ages and both sexes combined. An alphabetic index of included diagnoses as well as definitions of Hospital Groups appear on the following pages.

"The format in this study differs from prior Profile presentations. A single diagnosis is shown on each page, giving the number of cases, average stay and minimum-maximum stay tolerance range for patients grouped by age (under 65, 65+, and all ages combined), sex and Hospital Group. Data for each Hospital Group are shown in adjacent columns for ready comparison . . . ."

30. SAHAI, HARDEO; and JAMES E. VENEY. The estimation of inpatient stay parameters. *Inquiry* 4(1):44–67, March, 1967.

"The purpose of this paper is to provide a list of sample sizes necessary for making estimates of various aspects of the length of hospital stay for these diagnoses with specified degrees of accuracy." "The sample sizes listed are useful to the extent that they show the number of cases in a given diagnostic category which must be examined before an estimate of a certain precision can be made." The tables presented in this paper were compiled from 1965 New Jersey Blue Cross Plan data, which represent both a population and a sample. The data comprised length-of-stay distributions by 44 three-digit ICDA classifications of diseases, further subdivided into cases treated medically, cases treated surgically, and cases of persons under age 65 and those 65 and over. Four tables are presented. "The first is concerned with average length of stay, the second with 90th percentile of stays, the third gives sample sizes for relative precision in estimating the 90th percentile of stays, and the last shows sample sizes necessary for estimating other parameters of stay." The authors caution that their figures rest on acceptance of the assumption that a "sequential selection of all cases for a given diagnosis up to the necessary number of cases for a specific estimate about length of stay represents a probability sample of all cases yet to come." They also advise that accurate estimates require a large number of cases and cannot be done over a short period of time for small hospitals.

31. WOLFE, HARVEY. A computerized screening device for selecting cases for utilization review. *Medical Care* 5(1):44–51, January–February, 1967.

This study represents an exploratory effort into techniques of selecting cases for utilization review by the application of advanced statistical and data-processing methods. The approach presented makes use of regression analysis to predict an expected length of stay based upon a number of accessible factors, and then applies statistical control techniques to choose cases which have a high likelihood of being interesting to case reviewers. Dependent variables relating to the patient, to aspects of care, and to the particular hospital, and independent variables with any relationship to the independent variable were entered into a large multiple regression analysis. In a study of 841 cases of biliary tract surgery, five variables which explained over 80 per cent of the total variation in length of stay were used. Statistical control procedures based upon the concept of confidence limits were applied. Three cases of 28 days each were used to illustrate the system. Validation of acceptance or rejection by the system is accomplished by submitting a sample of both to a panel of physicians who make a decision with the use of the medical record.

Appropriateness of Utilization

32. BROWNING, FRANCIS E. "The Record in Hospital Bed Utilization." In *Utilization Review: A Handbook for the Medical Staff.* Chicago: American Medical Association, 1965, p. 77–82.

To explore the extent of agreement among physicians making judgments from records, the Medical Society of the County of Monroe undertook a three-month study of a random sample of surgical discharges in seven hospitals. Each of 1,763 records was examined independently by two physicians for instances of poor utilization. A questionnaire was used, the first part of which was prepared by the record librarian. Each physician reviewed records in his own hospital and at least one other hospital. The first and second sets of observations were tabulated to determine the extent of agreement between the two observer groups. The preliminary results disclose only 20 percent agreement between reviewing physicians for instances of improper utilization. There was higher agreement (31 percent) where delay between admission and surgery was deemed improper, and less agreement (3.7 percent) on the delay in providing consultation or X-ray services. The article speculates that perhaps hospital records are unsuitable in their present form to provide information germane to utilization.

33. CRISTO, CARMEN. 'Surveyor opinion' development and implementation in Monroe County, New York. *J. Amer. Med. Assoc.* 196(12):1065–1066, June 20, 1966.

An account of several studies spearheaded by the Monroe County Medical Society's Coordinating Committee on Utilization, using "observer teams" to survey records to guarantee efficient and effective use. One study of seven local general hospitals, using both a team from within the hospital and a team from outside, found close agreement between the two (14 percent and 18 percent respectively) on inappropriate use. Another study of 1,763 records, each reviewed independently by two observers for appropriateness of diagnostic admission and shorter stay, showed good agreement between the two surveyors (average of 10.9 percent for inappropriate utilization). Still a third study used two observers who reviewed the chart only and two who were free to tap any or all other sources of information. Again, 10.6 percent and 10.9 percent inappropriate utilization was recorded.

34. FITZPATRICK, THOMAS B.; DONALD C. RIEDEL; and BEVERLY C. PAYNE. Character and Effectiveness of Hospital Use: Project 2. In McNerney, Walter. *Hospital and Medical Economics.* Chicago: Hospital Research and Educational Trust, 1962, pp. 361–592.

To define the total picture of proper and improper hospital use, a collection and analysis of data on patient characteristics, services rendered, charges for same, and environmental factors was undertaken. 10,935 discharges during the year 1958 from a sample of hospitals were studied. Age, sex, diagnostic category, and services rendered were detailed and interrelated. The latter included information on operations performed, length of stay, number of discharges in 1958, and ancillary services expressed as weighted values in terms of units derived from a relative value scale. Charges for services and the source of payment were also considered a potential influence on utilization. The environmental factors analyzed were hospital characteristics—size, scope of service, medical staff—and physician characteristics, specialty status.

Measurement of hospital use was made by developing criteria by diagnosis, which was done by panels of physicians. For 18 diagnoses, (from records of 5,750 cases), indications for admission, hospital services required, expected length of stay, complications that may extend stay, and implications for discharge were established. In addition, the attending physician was interviewed to determine nonmedical factors involved, and the influence of such factors as cost. The authors state 11 detailed conclusions from the study and make specific recommendations for improvement. The entire discourse is supported by many and detailed tables presenting multiple cross tabulations.

Appendices give methodological and technical details for:
Diagnostic Categories; Distribution of Sampled Discharges
Criteria of Effectiveness of Hospital Use
Forms Used in Gathering Data
Probability Samples of Michigan Hospitals
Sampling Within Hospitals
Estimation Procedures; Sampling Variability
Projection of Hospital Admission Rate for Michigan
Selected Comparisons of Estimates from Projects 1 (Population Survey) and 2 (Hospital Use).

35. GREENBERG, SIDNEY M.; and THERESA ROGERS. Study uncovers "unnecessary" long-term stays in a short-term hospital. *Hospitals* 41(21):76,78,80, 82, November 1, 1967.

At the New York Hospital-Cornell Medical Center, during the year 1961, a sample of 195 of 612 long-term patients, representing 86 medical and surgical physicians, was selected for study. The physicians were queried as to the patients' potential for earlier discharge and given a list of various extended-care facilities for consideration. From the physician evaluations it was determined that 10 percent of the total bed days used by this group of patients could have been saved. Twenty-eight percent of the patients could have been discharged earlier. The physicians' further comments on the need for other types of facilities are presented.

36. RIEDEL, D. C. and T. B. FITZPATRICK. *Patterns of Patient Care.* Ann Arbor: University of Michigan, 1964.

(Publisher's Summary) This monograph is based on an extended analysis of data from the study of the "Character and Effectiveness of Hospital Use," one of the thirteen projects in the University of Michigan Study of Hospital and Medical Economics conducted at the behest of the Governor's Study Commission on Prepaid Hospital and Medical Care Plans, and published as the two-volume Hospital and Medical Economics in 1962 by the Hospital Research and Educational Trust of the American Hospital Association.

The data for the Michigan Study were derived from the medical and financial records of a probability sample of discharges from Michigan hospitals. Panels of medical specialists established criteria in 18 diagnostic categories for appropriateness of admission, for length of stay, and for the use of hospital services such as X-ray and laboratory procedures. These criteria for appropriate use of the hospital were compared with the actual care received by the patients in the selected diagnostic categories. In a subsample of cases, interviews were conducted with the attending physician in order to elicit unrecorded medical and extra-medical information which might have affected the doctor's decision regarding the patient's care.

From among the 18 diagnoses examined in the original study, Riedel and Fitzpatrick have selected six which appear frequently as causes of admission to the hospital: appendicitis, fibromyoma of the uterus, cholecystitis and cholelithiasis, urinary tract infection, diabetes mellitus, and acute myocardial infarction. The purpose of the authors is to study factors influencing variation in hospital use and the effectiveness of use in greater depth than was possible in the original study. The explanatory variables employed are selected patient, physician, and hospital characteristics which appeared to be important determinants of utilization in the earlier analyses. The principal analytic tool employed in the present study is the multivariate technique first used in the Population Survey of the Michigan Study, allowing the authors to appraise the relative influence of the selected variables on hospital use. Nearly all of the tabulations contained in this monograph were not reported in the earlier publication.

The present analysis is prefaced by a discussion of previous studies of hospital utilization as well as an analytical framework for evaluating the methodologies of such studies . . . .

Chapter I describes characteristics of the patients in each of the selected diagnostic categories and the characteristics of the hospitals and physicians providing the care. Chapter III describes variation in hospital use according to such measures as length of stay, units of diagnostic X-ray and units of laboratory procedures, and relates this variation to patient and provider characteristics, e.g., whether complications were recorded, qualifications of medical staff, sex of patient. Chapter IV discusses how effectively the hospitals were used and gives an analysis of the factors associated with inappropriate admissions, overstay, and understay.

The appendices contain the specifics of the major methodological techniques used in the study and some detailed tabulations which are only summarized in body of the text. Appendix A briefly describes the overall sampling plan employed to represent the population of discharges from Michigan hospitals during 1958. Appendix B discusses the multivariate analytic technique used in this study, and provides the detailed tabulations resulting from these analyses; the reader interested in pursuing the detailed relationships highlighted in the following chapters will find these tabulations most useful. Appendix C describes in detail the criteria for effective use of the hospital, for the six diagnoses under consideration in this report developed by the panels of medical specialists and provides a list of the panel members. Appendix D contains several tabulations not directly used in the text but useful to any reader interested in gaining additional insight into the nature of the basic distributions of length of stay by various patient, physician, and hospital characteristics; it also includes additional information about a few basic relationships between patient and provider characteristics.

37. SLEE, VERGIL N. "Uniform Methods of Measuring Utilization." In *Nat'l Conference on Utilization* (March 2–3, 1962). Report Series #2. Chicago: American Hospital Association, 1962.

The author sets forth requisites for measuring utilization: presence of something to measure; a rule or yardstick; and adequate information system (which is dependent upon the medical record). He describes the Professional Activity Study and the Medical Audit Program as a means of bridging the gap between gross statistics and patients' charts. Measurement of the first of three aspects of the patient's story, the appropriateness of the hospitalization, he describes with comparison among five hospitals of 1,000 medical cases. Length of stay he illustrates from PAS figures on tonsillectomies in two hospitals with mention of the reasons found for variation, and with a table showing all PAS pneumonia cases in 1963. Other PAS statistics are presented to demonstrate variation among individual physicians in one hospital, comparison between one doctor and the average for all others, and interhospital comparisons. Also included are PAS figures to illustrate the third aspect of the patient's story—utilization of hospital services.

38. ZIMMER, JAMES G. An evaluation of observer variability in a hospital bed utilization study. *Medical Care* 5(4):221–233, July–August, 1967.

(Author summary) A study of the methodology of general hospital bed utilization review is described in which the main focus is on the variability in observer opinions.

Teams of four physician observers, working in a university general hospital, made independent observations on randomly selected beds, the major decision being on the appropriateness of the current occupancy.

Agreement between observers was only slightly improved when information additional to that in the hospital charts was made available through patient and staff interview, and there was a tendency among those observers to decide more often that the bed occupancy was appropriate.

While there was no significant difference between the utilization decisions made by full-time medical school staff and part-time private practicing physician observers on the Medical and Surgical services, the full-time observers on the Pediatric and Gynecology services decided that beds were being inappropriately utilized significantly more frequently than did the part-time observers on those services.

Overall agreement between all four observers on appropriateness of utilization was fairly good (75 percent), but specific agreement was poor on the patients whom one or more observers considered to be inappropriately utilizing, all four agreeing on only 1.7 percent of those, three or more out of four on 4.5 percent, two or more on 10.0 percent, and one or more on 26.6 percent.

Four general characteristics (duration of hospitalization, age, status, and duration of stay post-operation) of the patients studied correlated positively with the observer decision that Utilization was inappropriate, but all of these factors may not be independent variables.

The difficulties in arriving at exact utilization statistics and the problems of variability of observer opinion are discussed in the light of the results, and a general view of the objectives and methodology of utilization studies is presented.

Physician Performance and the Process of Care

39. BEAUMONT, GRAHAM; DAVID FEIGAL; RICHARD M. MAGRAW; EDWARD C. DEFOE; JAMES B. CAREY. Medical auditing in a comprehensive clinic program. *J. Med. Ed.* 42(4):359–367, April, 1967.

    The clinic program at the University of Minnesota Medical School assigns the role of responsible physician in management of outpatients to the senior student. Patients are randomly assigned and charts are randomly selected for audit, which takes place six weeks after a patient's initial visit. The audit committee is composed of four students and two staff members. The diagnostic, chart-recording, and management deficiencies found as a result of audit are discussed in this paper. Two tests of validity were applied, one of which resulted in the formulation of a spot-check questionnaire. The limitations of this audit, its usefulness as an educational tool, and the role of the family doctor in the program are presented.

40. CLUTE, KENNETH F. "The Quality of General Practice." In *The General Practitioner.* Toronto: University of Toronto Press, 1963. Chapters 16, 17, 18.

    Clute reports on a survey study instituted by the College of General Practice of Canada designed to assess the quality of care rendered by general practitioners in Ontario and Nova Scotia. These three chapters focus on assessment methodology and results. Physician observers watched licensed practitioners in the office, home, and hospital for three days, after which the practitioners were assigned points on the basis of criteria, previously formulated by Peterson, which consisted of the following major categories (each with subheadings): history-taking, elements of physical examination, laboratory work, therapy, preventive medicine, and record quality. Only items on which at least 80 percent of the physicians were able to be assessed were retained on the rating scale, and physicians were eligible for rating only when treating the following cases: (1) new patients, (2) patients with new illnesses, (3) patients requesting an examination, or (4) patients whose appearance or complaint indicated the need for care. Scores were expressed as a percentage of the total number of points that were assignable for items on which that particular doctor could be assessed. Practitioners were also classified into five groups based on an overall opinion of the physician observers regarding their practice quality. Results are presented in terms of both the criteria enumerated and appropriate referrals made. When quality of practice was cross-tabulated with other factors the following emerged: quality of practice decreased as the physician became older; high medical-school grades were found among those practicing a higher quality of medicine.

41. COWLES, JOHN T. A critical-comments approach to the rating of medical students' clinical performance. *J. Med. Educ.* 40(2):188–198, February, 1965.

This study derives from the Clinical Performance Record (CPR) developed at the University of Pittsburgh and in use since 1956. A CPR form is completed for each student on medical service. Evaluations of all third- and fourth-year students in three successive calendar years (85 in each) are reported here. 2,300 instructor comments were abstracted and sorted into eight categories, e.g., Knowledge and Understanding, Rapport with Patients. Ten senior internists rated the comments on a 6-point scale of goodness. Also 11 nonphysicians did the same rating. The mean and standard deviation of ratings for each comment were computed separately for the physicians and the nonphysicians. The content of the comments, frequency distribution of comments by scale value, the proportion of comments in each category, the reliability of the comments (interjudge agreement), and the comparison of comments on third- and fourth-year students are discussed. Suggestions for future studies are made.

42. DENTON, JOHN C.; AMASA B. FORD; RALPH E. LISKE; and ROBERT S. ORT. Predicting judged quality of patient care in general hospitals. *Hlth. Servs. Res.* 2 (1):26–33, Spring, 1967.

(Journal Summary) Cleveland physicians with in-depth knowledge about hospitals in their community were asked to rank general hospitals, on a 5-point scale, in an attempt to evaluate quality of patient care. Nine physicians showed reasonable agreement in their judgments. In a broader sample, six additional physicians ranked the same hospitals to provide a check on overall inter-rater reliability. Average hospital rank assigned by the first group correlated $+.89$ with average rank for the broader samples, indicating good criterion reliability.

Later, published data about the hospitals, such as number of residency programs offered, number of beds, and average length of stay, were correlated with the rankings provided by all 15 physicians. Resulting correlations were substantial (e.g., $+.86$ for number of approved residency programs), and the best combination of three variables predicted the criterion with a multiple correlation of $+.94$. Cross validation in four other metropolitan areas in Ohio and Pennsylvania, where 75 physician raters provided ratings of 36 general hospitals, showed that the three variables isolated for the Cleveland sample predicted the overall quality of patient care in the four other communities, with a correlation of $+.82$.

The study was made by a team of physicians and psychologists as part of a larger investigation of practicing physicians and the doctor-patient relationship. The work reported here was directed at establishing ratings of the hospitals in which these physicians work and were trained.

43. EHRLICH, J.; M. A. MOREHEAD; and R. E. TRUSSELL. *The Quantity, Quality and Costs of Medical and Hospital Care Secured by a Sample of Teamster Families in the New York Area.* New York: Columbia University School of Public Health and Administrative Medicine, 1960, 83pp.

This study was undertaken, at the request of the Teamsters Joint Council 16 and Management Hospitalization Trust Fund, to analyze factors relating to the cost and quality of medical and hospital care secured by Teamsters and their families. The sample was selected from individuals with specific diagnoses who had a claim paid by Blue Cross during the last six months of 1959 (406 admissions to 100 hospitals). The study had two major components, a household survey and a medical audit. Selected families were interviewed about financial aspects of their medical care, doctors they consulted, insurance coverage and use, and an opinion of their personal overall medical care. Information was gathered on number of physicians, cost to hospital, charges previous to, as well as during, hospital stay, number of physician visits. The other part of this study concerned a medical audit from photostatic copies of hospital records made by specialists recognized as experts in the disease for which the patient was hospitalized. Type of hospital used, length of stay, type of illness, estimate of the necessity for hospitalization, and a judgment of care received were studied, the latter in accordance with the way the judging physician would have managed the case and rated as excellent, good, fair, and poor. Results of the analysis of costs of medical care showed considerable out-of-pocket medical expenses for the Teamsters, while the analysis of the surveyor's review of the hospital admissions showed that there were many problems relating to quality medical care which overshadowed problems of unnecessary use of hospitals. The report includes: (1) demographic description of patients, their patterns of medical care, hospital and patient costs, and charges in relation to length of stay; (2) results of the audit with case summaries as examples, and illustrations of each level of rated care—excellent, good, fair, poor. Qualifications of the attending physicians are also detailed. Data are presented in numerous tables (see also entry 50).

44. FALK, I. S.; H. K. SCHONFELD; B. R. HARRIS; S. J. LANDAU; and S. S. MILES. The development of standards for the audit and planning of medical care I. Concepts, research design, and the content of primary physicians' care. *Amer. J. Pub. Hlth.* 57(7):1118–1136, July, 1967.

> The question "what should be done for the prevention, diagnosis, therapy, and aftercare of people having various diseases and disorders" is the focus of this study, which develops standards for the content of good clinical performance in quantitative terms. Comprehensiveness is intended as to conditions requiring care and to the kinds of care required for a general population, first from a primary physician and then from a referral specialist as indicated. Structured interviews were conducted with 36 internists and 21 pediatricians, all in private practice with faculty appointments, and 230 disease categories were defined. In addition, a narrative description of the disease was provided by the interviewed physician. The results were composited and the completed narrative extended by data from the schedules. The quantitative data were coded and tabulated, providing tentative standards in the forms of totals, averages, and distributions. This paper concerns itself only with the role of the primary physician in care of adults and illustrates the method of "index standards of needed care" with seven tables (using 18 selected diagnoses): visits needed for a specific disease; distribution of patients by number of diagnostic visits; time required for first diagnostic visit; distribution of patients with a specific disease by number of visits for diagnosis, treatment, and/or follow-up; distribution of patients by type of referral specialist for diagnosis; distribution of patients by days of hospitalization under the care of the primary physician. In addition, the authors discuss applications of the data to the clinical audit, and in national estimates of medical care resources and costs.

45. GEORGOPOULOS, BASIL S.; and FLOYD C. MANN. *The Community General Hospital.* New York: Macmillan, 1962. Chapters 5, 8.

> From 10 participating hospitals, similar in size, type, and administrative structure, the authors developed four measures of patient care: an overall measure; a medical care measure; a nursing care measure; and a comparative overall measure.
>
> Nursing care measure. Medical staff, registered nurses, lab and X-ray technicians, the administrator, nonmedical department heads, and the trustee executive committee at each hospital answered the question, "How good is the nursing care given to patients in this hospital?" Seven alternate choices were given for the respondent to check, ranging from outstanding to poor. Means for each group within one hospital, and then the combined means for all groups in each hospital were computed. The hospitals were then rank ordered by means. Intercorrelations among the four groups and all groups combined revealed the nursing care measure to be "stable and reliable." This measure was tested for validity against volunteered comments from nonrespondents, data about the composition of the nursing staff, and auxiliary opinions about how well the nursing staff performed its job.
>
> Medical care measure. This was derived in much the same way as the nursing care measure, except that the respondents to the question,

BIBLIOGRAPHY

"How good would you say is the medical care given to patients in this hospital?" were only physicians, and that more weight was given to the responses from physicians in certain key positions. Internal consistency of this measure was found to be quite high, and validity was tested with information obtained from 7 other sources, including ratings by outside doctors and mortality rates obtained from medical records.

Overall patient care measure. The same respondents as in the nursing care measure answered the question, "How would you rate the quality of the overall care that patients receive from this hospital?" The computation of means was likewise similar. Also, this measure was examined for consistency among the subgroups of respondents, and it was validated against "customer satisfaction" data and community reputation indicators.

Comparative overall patient care measure. "How would you rate the quality of overall patient care in this hospital as compared to similar other community hospitals?" was asked of the same respondents as in the nursing care and overall patient care measures. This measure also proved stable and internally consistent and was validated by comparing it with the other three measures.

Finally, the authors analyzed the relationships among the four measures.

In Chapter 8 the authors report their findings in relating the four measures of patient care to other aspects of hospitals. These variables were studied by correlation analysis and are as follows: the relative adequacy of various material facilities; hospital income and expenditures; certain size-related aspects; skill composition and distribution of nursing and medical staffs; absenteeism and turnover among nursing personnel; organizational coordination; aspects of intraorganizational strain; complementarity of expectations between the medical staff and the nursing staff; medical committee activity and performance; and performance of paramedical departments. "Stated in their most general (and of necessity least precise) form, the principal findings from this part of the study show that the quality of patient care in the participating hospitals is

not higher in institutions having
    superior material facilities
    better financial status or higher income
    higher costs or higher expenses
    more personnel or a larger paid staff
    larger size in terms of number of beds and patient admissions
    medical committees individually performing at a high level

but *is inversely (negatively)* related to
    the level of prevailing tension among interacting groups and departments in the organization
    the rate of unexcused absenteeism among professional nurses
    the degree of experienced "unreasonable" pressure for better performance by nonmedical personnel
        by nonmedical personnel

and *positively* related to
    the quality of organizational coordination in the hospital
    coordination within the nursing department alone

certain aspects of the composition and distribution of the therapeutic staff (medical and nursing staff)

the performance of the nursing department (but not the individual performance of the records, laboratory, and X-ray departments)

complementarity of work-related expectations between doctors and nurses

the rate of turnover among nurse's aides."

46. HELFER, RAY E. Estimating the quality of patient care in a pediatric emergency room. *J. Med. Educ.* 42(3):224–248, March, 1967.

This study was based on concepts described by Williamson (entry 60). At the University of Colorado Medical Center a chart-review was done over a two-month period, in three phases, by the author, on all children presenting with cough, cold, or fever. Baseline data were obtained from the work of the two interns staffing the emergency room, after which there were chart review sessions with full professors. A second survey was done followed by a discussion of the study in detail, and then a third survey was made. Proficiency Index, Efficiency Index, and Competence Index computed in the three different phases revealed little improvement as a result of the chart review, but "dramatic" changes after the interns were acquainted with what was expected of them.

47. HUBBARD, JOHN P.; EDITHE J. LEVITT; CHARLES F. SCHUMACHER; and TRUMAN SCHNABEL. An objective evaluation of clinical competence. *New Engl. J. Med.* 272(25):1321–1328, June 24, 1965.

The National Board of Medical Examiners, in cooperation with the American Institute for Research, undertook a two-year study to devise a means of evaluating such components of medical skill as history-taking, detection and interpretation of significant signs and symptoms, diagnostic acumen, and judgment in treatment. The first step—to define clinical competence—was approached by the "critical-incident" technique. About 600 senior physicians and residents reported by interview and questionnaire 3,300 incidents about the performance of interns ("good" and "poor"). These incidents were classified into nine major areas to evaluate. An effort to improve the reliability of the bedside-observation method of evaluation proved unsuccessful and the method was discarded. The three methods adopted and used are described in detail: (1) a motion picture film of an undiagnosed patient accompanied by multiple-choice questions on the case; (2) simultaneous presentation of several pictorial reproductions of clinical material with accompanying questions requiring discrimination in differential diagnosis; (3) "programmed testing" which simulates the clinic situation. Reliability of these measures was tested by comparing two scores and was achieved to the degree of 0.87. By subjective judgment the examiners considered the test to be valid, and independence correlations of this test to parts I and II of the board examinations proved to be positive, though moderate.

48. JUNGFER, C. C.; and J. M. LAST. Clinical performance in Australian general practice. *Medical Care* 2(2):71–83, April–June, 1965.

A study based on the design used by Peterson *et al.* in North Carolina, using physician observers. One hundred eight visited practitioners, who were selected to represent various styles of practice—urban and rural—and who provided the data (including questionnaire information). A structured checklist and a five-point rating scale were used. History-taking was evaluated by the methods used by both Peterson and Clute. Scores were expressed as percentages of their possible maxima. Performance of the whole sample of physicians regarding separate components of their work is discussed and shown in tables. Information about the physicians' graduate training was related to their clinical performance. The authors discuss implications of the findings about examinations and treatment and about the professional education of physicians.

49. LEMBCKE, PAUL; and OLIVE G. JOHNSON. *A Medical Audit Report.* Los Angeles: University of California, 1963, 291pp.

"Comparison of the findings in a 200-bed suburban hospital with those in university teaching hospitals . . . also, the findings before and after a continuing medical audit was established in a large community hospital." The study hospital contracted for an audit by the author, who reviewed all cases audited and abstracted records of fatal cases. Two medical record librarians abstracted all other records. Evaluations were made according to "objective criteria where such existed or could be formulated." Then comparison was made with results of applying the same method in a university teaching hospital. In many types of surgery, comparisons were made with three teaching hospitals and one community hospital. The *Report* includes an analysis and discussion of all deaths by case. A list of criteria for female pelvic surgery is given. Then the cases studied for each of 15 areas of medicine and surgery (24 medical conditions, 19 surgical procedures, and obstetrics) are summarized in comparison with the control-hospital cases. Each case is listed as justified or unjustified, with pertinent facts; the significant features considered in the evaluation are discussed.

50. MOREHEAD, M. A. et al. *A Study of the Quality of Hospital Care Secured by a Sample of Teamster Family Members in New York City.* New York: Columbia University School of Public Health and Administrative Medicine, 1964, 98pp.

The second of two studies completed by the Medical Audit Unit of the Teamster Center Program jointly sponsored by the Hospitalization Trust Fund, Montefiore Hospital, and the Columbia University School of Public Health and Administrative Medicine. The present report is a study of the quality of medical care received by, and the necessity for hospitalization of a sample of patients who had a claim paid by Blue Cross in May 1962 to hospitals in New York City. Four hundred thirty admissions (292 patients) from 98 different New York City hospitals and among nine different specialty fields were in the final study. "A random sample, stratified by the Welfare Fund, was made of all claims, with the exception of those for normal deliveries and tonsillectomies and adenoidectomies, which were excluded from the original request. Other hospital admissions experienced by the sample patients during a five-year study period surrounding the admission under study were also included.

"Based upon written consents, photostatic copies of the hospital records of 78 percent of the original sample were obtained. The records were reviewed by thirteen clinicians with recognized professional standing in their specialties. The surveyors were asked to judge on the basis of their knowledge and experience the quality of the medical care rendered and the necessity for hospitalization. In order to assess the reproducibility of evaluation results, two surveyors independently reviewed each record in the major fields of medicine, surgery, and pediatrics—67 percent of all admissions reviewed."

Percentage of admissions which received "optimal" care and of those considered "necessary" was considered in relation to the kind of hospital and to the qualifications of the attending physician. The report details characteristics of the hospitals and considers the relationship of the "optimal" and "necessary" admissions to the type of hospital, the classification of the physician, and to the medical specialty. Differences in opinion between surveyors are detailed by case. Case summaries, comparisons of surveyors' opinions, and tables are included (also see entry 43).

51. PETERSON, O. L.; and E. BARSAMIAN. "Diagnostic Performance." In Jacquez, J. A. (Ed). *The Diagnostic Process.* Ann Arbor: The University of Michigan, 1963, pp. 347–362.

This paper deals with a method to measure certain aspects of the quality of surgical care. On a population drawn from the O. R. register, appendectomies, cholecystectomies, and pelvic surgery were studied, though only the latter is reported here. Ten "processes" or parts of a complete evaluation of a patient's condition were graded and coded: completeness of history; completeness of physical examination; symptoms plus findings plus laboratory data = diagnosis; symptoms plus findings plus laboratory data = justified surgery; diagnosis = pathology; specificity of surgery; clinical pathology = pathology; appraisal of tissue; postoperative care; complications. An example of fibroids is used to give the following tables with a discussion of each: symptoms that must be considered in fibroids; symptoms that might be expected in postmenopausal patients; physical examination; the process in which the relation of workup and diagnosis are examined; relationship between symptoms, findings, and laboratory; indications for surgery; minimal pathology consistent with symptoms. The Stein-Leventhal Syndrome is also given as an example. The rest of the article is devoted to showing how it is possible to categorize a specific illness in relation to findings plus current knowledge of the disease process. The authors feel that this type of grading and coding system is applicable for computers and could take over some of the functions of a review committee in the future.

52. PETERSON, OSLER L.; ERNEST M. BARSAMIAN; and MURRAY EDEN. A study of diagnostic performance: a preliminary report. *J. Med. Educ.* 41 (8): 797–803, August, 1966.

A study of surgical diagnosis was designed to formulate a system of measuring surgical performance and to determine the relationship between hospital training and surgical skills. This report covers only pelvic surgery. Relationships between symptoms and diagnoses were outlined in a logic tree, which aided gynecologists in defining their systematic approach to two of the processes involved in a hospital episode, making the diagnosis and deciding to do surgery. A computer program was then written which was used as a diagnostic machine. The type of errors encountered in an experience with 48 patients who had hysterectomies is discussed. The authors emphasize that the computer failures were mainly related to poor information or failure to record data vital to the decision-making process.

53. PRICE, PHILIPS B.; CALVIN, W. TAYLOR; JAMES M. RICHARDS; and TONY L. JACOBSEN. Measurement of physician performance. *J. Med. Educ.* 39(2): 203–211, February, 1964.

From records, questionnaires, and interviews, personal and professional information was collected about 102 full-time faculty members, 190 urban specialists, 110 urban general practitioners, and 105 rural general practitioners. Grades in college and medical school were included. Two hundred different measures of performance were thus identified, not all of which were common to all four groups of physicians. Eighty measures (limited by computer analysis) were studied for each group. The measures were converted to scores, degree of relationship between each measure was computed, and factor analysis was applied. Clusters of relatively independent variables were isolated and a profile of performance was derived. Examples are given. By examining the 849 intercorrelations of measures of academic achievement and of performance in practice, it was shown that formal education grade points are "almost completely independent of all factors having to do with performance as a physician."

54. RICHARDSON, F. MACD. Rochester region perinatal study. *N.Y.J. Med.* 67(9):1205–1210, May 1, 1967.

In summary, a sample of complicated deliveries within hospitals in the Rochester Hospital Service Region was examined by peer judgments solicited from three other areas of the state. Judgments were first made independently by two reviewers of hospital charts of the mothers and babies involved. Judgments of care were made using the terms "satisfactory" or "unsatisfactory." All "unsatisfactory" judgments and a sample of "satisfactory" agreements between the two reviewers were in turn reviewed by a three-man panel within each appropriate specialty. "Application of a panel 'correction factor' to the total of paired reviewer opinions resulted in a final judgment of 'satisfactory' in 77.5 percent of the deliveries reviewed and in 79.5 percent of the care provided to the resulting newborn infants."

The paper also presents results of additional comments made by the reviewers regarding the care rendered.

55. SCHONFELD, HYMAN K.; ISIDORE S. FALK; PAUL H. LAVIETES; SAUL MILES; and JACK S. LANDAU. The development of standards for the audit and planning of medical care: pathways among primary physicians and specialists for diagnosis and treatment. *Medical Care* 6(2):101–114, March–April, 1968.

This paper reports a continuation of the research outlined in entry 44. The term *pathway* denotes the "sequence of medical services and their proper time order." This stage of the project included opinions of specialist physicians and makes use of interview schedules similar to those described in the above-mentioned basic paper, with a specific disease as a starting point. For this present report, three diseases are used to illustrate the methodology in tabulating and presenting the kinds of physicians required for major pathways. Implications of the differences in opinions among the primary and referral physicians are discussed. The authors state that data are not available to measure the effect of a given pathway on the health of a patient, but that estimates of needed personnel and facilities and cost per unit of service can be determined.

56. SCHONFELD, H. K.; I. S. FALK; H. R. SLEEPER; and W. D. JOHNSTON. The content of good dental care: methodology in a formulation for clinical standards and audits, and preliminary findings. *Amer. J. Pub. Hlth.* 57(7):1137–1146, July, 1967.

This paper reports on the dental portion of an overall content-of-care study done at Yale University School of Medicine. Methodology, therefore, is similar to that reported in item 44.

57. SPARLING, J. FREDERICK. Measuring medical care quality: A comparative study. Part I. *Hospitals* 36(7):62, 64, 67–8, March 16, 1962.

Part I examines the percentage of necessary appendectomies in two teaching and three community hospitals in Baltimore. One thousand and two patients who had primary appendectomy surgery in 1957 and 1958 were studied. The study focused on an "efficiency factor," the necessary appendectomies as percentage of the total performed. A chi square test proved the combined efficiency factor for the university hospitals to be significantly greater than that for community hospitals at the 1 percent level. Necessary appendectomies in the university hospital totaled 67.3 percent, and 49.2 percent in the community hospital. Data on six possible variables are given: accommodation, pay status, age, sex, completeness of examination, and race. Males, nonwhites, and those with a good examination had a significantly higher number of necessary appendectomies; patients with Blue Cross of prepayment plan in community hospitals had a significantly higher number of unnecessary appendectomies than private or welfare patients (see entry 58 for Part II).

58. SPARLING, J. FREDERICK. Measuring medical care quality: a comparative study. Part II. *Hospitals* 36(7):56–57, 60–61, April 1, 1962.

Length of patient stay, number of X-rays, laboratory tests, and drug usage are discussed as part of quality care evaluation, and also whether there is an optimum amount of service consistent with good-quality medical care. From data on appendectomies done in university and community hospitals, a frequency curve and computation of median length of stay showed a difference of one and one-half days and two days respectively between the hospitals, length of stay being shorter for the university hospitals. X-ray charges and use of antibiotics are compared in relation to the variables, room service, insurance coverage, sex, race, and age. Use of antibiotics was less in a university hospital for the same type of disease; ward patients in university hospitals had much higher drug utilization and much less X-ray utilization than did private patients. Patients with the shortest lengths of stay and most visits to hospital were those who had insurance coverage. As age increased so did length of stay. The author includes a discussion of the limitations of the study (see entry 57 for Part I).

BIBLIOGRAPHY

59. STAPLETON, JOHN F.; and JAMES A. ZWERNEMAN. The influence of an intern-resident staff on the quality of private patient care. *J. Amer. Med. Assoc.* 194(8):877–882, November 22, 1965.

This describes an effort at St. Vincent Hospital, Worcester, Massachusetts, to compare objectively the quality of medical care given to 1,356 elective admissions on two geographically separate private medical services, one a teaching (T) unit and one a nonteaching (NT) unit, and also among attending physicians in various categories in this single community hospital. Records of patients, 625 from the T service and 731 from the NT service, discharged between 11/1/62 and 4/30/64 were drawn on a "random and systematic" basis being dependent upon the record room's order of release of completed records. Records were grouped by service and subclassified by three categories of attending physicians: (1) group A—physicians certified by the American Board of Internal Medicine or the American College of Physicians; (2) group B—noncertified M.D.s graduated prior to 1945; and (3) noncertified physicians graduated since 1945. The Commission on Professional Activities Studies (PAS completed medical audits on alternate records, 204 from the T service and 235 from the NT service). The two patient populations were similar with respect to parameters such as age, sex, death rate, autopsy rate, diagnoses, and hospitalization costs. "Variety" and "Impact" indices devised by PAS facilitated comparisons between the two services as well as among the attending physician categories. Differences in favor of the T section were evident in several procedures. Certain trends appeared in the study: (1) teaching service generally seemed to provide more complete care than the nonteaching service; and (2) certified physicians seemed to provide a more completed workup than the noncertified. The authors hesitate to attach any arbitrary statements to their results as they were mindful of a lack of rigid standards in the medical care field.

60. WILLIAMSON, JOHN W. Assessing clinical judgment. *J. Med. Educ.* 40(2): 180–187, February, 1965.

A simulated patient-problem technique is described where a list of possible diagnostic and therapeutic interventions is presented to the physician. The selections made are compared with criteria developed by specialists who rated each item on a scale from "very helpful" to "very harmful." Two scores were established: An Efficiency Index—percentage of selections that were helpful; and a Proficiency Index—percentage of agreement with the criterion group. A combined Competence Index was then calculated. An example of this method administered to 232 practicing physicians for three diseases is presented and discussed.

End Results and Program Effectiveness

61. BUBECK, ROY G., JR.; MATTHEWS, JAMES G.; RIEMANN, MARTIN L.; and HARVEY C. ORTH, JR. Maternal mortality: report of ten-year study of patients under osteopathic care. *J. Amer. Osteop. Assn.* 67(12):379–395, December, 1967.

(Journal Summary) Statistics have been compiled on all maternal deaths occurring under osteopathic care in the State of Michigan in a

10-year period. In a series of 197,484 births, a total of 104 maternal deaths occurred, giving a maternal death rate of 5.27 per 10,000 live births. The number of direct obstetric deaths was 63, giving an obstetric death rate of 3.19 per 10,000 live births. These figures compare favorably with those from other maternal mortality studies reported in the literature. The major causes of death are analyzed for their clinical implication. It is noted that 60 of the deaths were judged avoidable or possibly avoidable, with the physician believed to be wholly or partially responsible in 83.3 percent of them. It is urged strongly that similar maternal mortality studies be carried out in other states, with the results used for the education of physicians and nurses.

62. CHIANG, C. L. *An Index to Health: Mathematical Models.* Series 2, #5, Vital and Health Statistics. U.S. Public Health Service, 1965, 19pp.

The Index of Health (H) for a given population is composed of three separate variables: the number of illnesses, their duration, and time lost due to death. Mathematical models showing probability distributions for each component are presented. The components may be viewed individually, for example, to forecast the number of illnesses an individual may expect in a given year, or the duration of illness. These two items taken together can give the expected total duration of illnesses within a given year. The author concludes with a warning that H is affected by population composition and he provides an adjustment formula.

63. GIBSON, COUNT D.; and BERNARD M. KRAMER. Site of care in medical practice. *Medical Care* 3(1):14–17, January–March, 1965.

A study was undertaken by the Tufts University School of Medicine at the Columbia Point Housing Development near Boston to evaluate the effect of site on the process of medical care. Using the Home Medical Care Service program previously established, an office was set up in the housing development, but equipment was the same type carried regularly on house calls, thus focusing on site of care as the independent variable. Home and office episodes were randomly chosen from incoming calls; such factors as socioeconomic status and previous medical care did not vary significantly between the two groups. Externs assigned to the project for a period of two months spent half their time at the project site and the other half on house call duty, thus serving as their own control. Data were grouped around three main areas of concern: (1) the illness and its treatment; (2) performance and subjective reaction of the externs; and (3) performance and subjective reactions of the mothers of pediatric patients. Three major sources for these data consisted of a questionnaire completed by extern, the medical record, and personal interview of a sample of 145 mothers. Results indicated that externs preferred the physical environment of the office but expressed greater satisfaction with selected aspects of the home setting, two of which were good rapport with mother, and opportunity for uncovering additional disease through the "encounter effect" of dealing directly with the family. No discernible differences were found with respect to extern performance. The data taken together indicated that site of care is a meaningful variable "in the effort to understand the reticular process of Medical Care."

BIBLIOGRAPHY

64. HAGNER, SAMUEL B.; VICTOR J. LOCIERO; and WILLIAM A. STEIGNER. Patient outcome in a comprehensive medicine clinic: its retrospective assessment and related variables. *Medical Care* 6(2):144–156, March, 1968.

> A group of 174 patients treated by senior medical students at the Temple University Medical Center Comprehensive Medicine Clinic were followed by an open-ended interview two to three years after treatment. A "before treatment" evaluation was first formulated from clinic notes, diagnostic-management conference reports, and student papers about each patient. With the focus on function and behavior as indicators of the patient's well-being, a rating scale of six points was developed by two raters. A third judge tested reliability of the scale by rating the same patients. Of the 174 patients, 125 were interviewed, six had died, and the remaining 43 nonrespondents were treated as a third type of outcome in the data analysis, in addition to the "improved" and "unimproved" groups. These outcome groups were studied in relation to: personal patient characteristics—e.g., race, age, church attendance; childhood factors; socioeconomic variables; selected treatment variables—i.e., prognosis, number of clinic visits, mode of disposition; patients' attitudes about treatment and outcome. The authors believe their findings suggest "that some of the critical variables of medical care lie in the area of the doctor-patient relationship."

65. KATZ, SIDNEY; BEVERLY A. JACKSON; MARJORIE W. JAFFEE; ARTHUR LITTELL; and CHARLES E. TURK. Multidisciplinary studies of illness in aged persons—VI: Comparison study of rehabilitated and nonrehabilitated patients with fracture of the hip. *J. Chron. Dis.* 15:979–984, Oct. 1962.

> This study was designed to assess the use of evaluation of patient function methods for comparative studies in the rehabilitation of patients with hip fractures. Study patients came from two sources: (1) all patients with a fracture of less than six months' duration admitted to Benjamin Rose Hospital, Cleveland, between September 1956 and June 1959; (2) patients with hip fractures admitted to Highland View Hospital between November 1958 and December 1959. The control group consisted of all patients from the staff-orthopedic service of University Hospitals of Cleveland and from the private practice of five orthopedic surgeons between November 1958 and December 1959. The 114 study patients had comprehensive rehabilitation treatment and were matched with the controls on six factors: sex; age; type of medical care (staff vs. private); type of residence prior to fracture; and level of independence in activities of daily living (ADL) prior to fracture (gauged by a previously devised 7-grade index). Only 25 of the original 65 untreated patients proved suitable for matching. Differences between the two groups in course of illness were measured in terms of mortality rates, ambulation and ADL functioning, the last two judged by the researchers based on previously devised scales.

66. KIDD, CECIL B. Misplacement of the elderly in hospital. *Brit. Med. J.* 11:1491–1495, December 8, 1962.

> In a study previous to this one, a group of 100 geriatric patients in a mental hospital and a geriatric unit in Belfast were assessed for physical and psychiatric disability; 24 percent and 34 percent from the two facilities were judged misplaced. The present study is a follow-up

examination of the consequences of misplacement of these 100 patients. "The misplaced patients had a higher mortality in hospital than was found among the correctly placed patients. This was so in both hospitals. Also, their mortality was higher than that of patients suffering from similar ailments who had been admitted to the proper unit. Among the survivors, the misplaced patients were less often discharged than correctly placed patients. These differences were not accounted for by differences in age or sex, or by the seriousness of the illnesses. Patients with mixed physical and mental disabilities did not have an especially bad prognosis. Misplacement itself seemed to be directly responsible for the poor outcome of the patients. Reasons for this poor outcome are discussed, and ways of avoiding misplacement are outlined."

67. KUTNER, BERNARD. "Modes of Treating the Chronically Ill." In *Symposium of Research in Long-Term Care.* Proceedings, St. Louis [Jewish Hospital of St. Louis], 1963, pp. 48–57.

Out of concern for the socially debilitating effects of long-term illness, a demonstration project was set up in 1960 by Albert Einstein College of Medicine to deal with developing a community method of treatment. The author proposes that "living potential" should dictate hospital therapy policy and may not be congruent with "rehabilitation potential." In a hospital-based physical rehabilitation program an experimental milieu therapy ward was set up adjacent to a conventional (control) treatment ward in a large municipal general hospital. Two hundred patients in the study were to be measured against a baseline group of 100 patients who had completed their hospital stay prior to the study. The experimental ward staff were indoctrinated in principles of milieu therapy; lower echelon staff were included in conferences. In this ward a patient organization for discussion and planning was formed; patients and staff conferred on problems; families were involved in the therapeutic process. A research policy committee considered patient-group-initiated recommendations; patients were given a large share in carrying out suggestions. Measurement of patient progress was made at admission, one month later, at discharge, and at three months and one year following discharge. The 33 instruments used in the study are not detailed in the paper, but covered physician status and progress, attitudinal changes, opinions and specific knowledge, functional performance, etc. Changes made in the experimental program and marked observable improvements are recounted, although preliminary data on 40 discharged patients (about half from each ward) show only a slight advantage for experimental patients in daily performance and a greater posthospital adjustment. Patients' increased capacity for rehabilitation was also supported by self-evaluation.

68. LAWTON, M. POWELL; MORTON WARD; and SILVIA YAFFEE. Indices of health in an aging population. *J. of Geront.* 22(3):334–342, July, 1967.

(Author Summary) A group of 97 female and 52 male apartment dwellers of ages 66–90 were given a physical examination and were rated on a variety of aspects of health by a physician. Subjects also rated their own health according to various criteria, and their health behavior was recorded for a period of one year. Aspects of health which were sampled by these measures included life-threatening quality, degree of functional disability, emotional status, and degree of pain. The 30 separate measures were intercorrelated and factor-analyzed in order to determine what some of the basic health factors might be. Factors entitled Disability, Self-Perceived Health, Consensual Awareness of Health Status, Physician-Rated Health, Self-Protective Health Behavior, and Subjective Discomfort appeared in both male and female groups. These factors represented among them relatively pure self-estimate and physician-rated factors, as well as more complex factors derived from a variety of sources of data and conceptual aspects of health.

69. LIPWORTH, L.; J. A. H. LEE; and J. N. MORRIS. Case-fatality in teaching and non-teaching hospitals 1956–1959. *Medical Care* 1(2):71–76, April–June, 1963.

This report, issued through the Social Medicine Research Unit, Medical Research Council, London Hospital, is an analysis of three years' statistics which show differences in case fatality of certain conditions between teaching and nonteaching hospitals. Case fatality rates in nonteaching hospitals for immediate admissions of conditions, such as peptic ulcer, appendicitis, hernia of abdominal cavity with obstruction, cholelithiasis, hyperplasia of prostate and skull injuries, were between one percent and five percent higher than in teaching hospitals; "other admissions" (transfers from other hospitals) for surgery showed similar rates (one percent to six percent). Reasons for the differences noted are suggested: teaching hospitals may give superior treatment; patients who go to nonteaching hospitals may be socially or otherwise at an initial disadvantage; teaching hospitals have more consultants; and the proportion of older patients is greater in nonteaching hospitals.

70. LOCKWARD, H. J.; GEORGE A. F. LUNDBERG; and M. E. ODOROFF. Effect of intensive care on mortality rate of patients with myocardial infarcts. *Pub. Hlth. Rep.* 78(8):655–661, August, 1963.

To obtain data on the effect of intensive care on patient recovery, a study of patients with myocardial infarcts (exclusive of those dying within 48 hours after admission) was undertaken at Manchester (Connecticut) Memorial Hospital. The study subjects were: (a) all patients (74) admitted 1955–1956 with an unequivocal diagnosis of myocardial infarction and treated under the conventional system, and (b) all patients (101) admitted with the same diagnosis 1958–1959 and treated in the ICU. Data were analyzed regarding age, sex, good or poor risk, mortality (excluding deaths within 48 hours to control for poor risks), and use of anticoagulant therapy. From weighted average differences and weighted variances of the average difference, the mortality rate for the conventionally treated patients showed 15 percent greater. Mortality rate was 28 percent lower with use of anticoagulants when effects of sex, age, risk and type of care were held constant.

71. MEDALIE, JACK H.; and KALMAN J. MANN. Evaluation of medical care: methodological problems in a 6-year followup of a family and community health center. *J. Chron. Dis.* 19(1):17–33, January, 1966.

The Family and Community Health Center at Kirajat Hayonel was established in January 1953 to serve a housing section of Jerusalem.

A high percentage of the occupants had chronic diseases and were in need of welfare services. The Center operated on the principles of extended family care, 24-hour service, coordination of community agencies, and continuity of care. For evaluating this program, the methods of before and after study, a control group comparison, and matched sample from national figures were not feasible and were rejected in favor of comparison of local figures with national ones on a "one-shot basis." Comparison of demographic data showed the study population "sufficiently similar" to the national. Mortality, morbidity for six conditions, and hospitalization were three variables studied. Also a subjective observation is reported with supporting descriptions of community cooperation, attitudes, and behavior. (Despite fewer physician visits than in other sick-fund populations, the health of the neighborhood was better.) Finally, the authors speculate on how close the Center came to accomplishing its goal.

72. MELTZER, LAWRENCE E. Coronary units can help decrease deaths. *Mod. Hospital.* 104(1):102, 104, January, 1965.

A prestudy survey of 761 patients with acute myocardial infarctions revealed that 47 percent of deaths occurring in this group were caused by arrhythmias, most of which, if detected and treated immediately, need not prove fatal. On this premise, in 1963, a specific program for intensive coronary care, supported by grants from the Public Health Service and the National Institutes of Health was begun in Presbyterian Hospital in Philadelphia. The program calls for (1) continuous cardiographic observation, and (2) a system to terminate arrhythmias immediately after occurrence. Therefore, a two-bed, self-sufficient unit was provided to observe patients during the critical first 72 hours after admission. Patients were assigned by a random method to the Program Unit. Additional patients were treated in normal facilities and thus provided a control group. Six nurses were trained in special techniques for this setting and to begin treatment themselves if a physician was delayed past the crucial two-minute period. For 200 patients followed thus far in the experimental unit, a 30 percent lower death rate was obtained. The author stresses the importance of the trained nursing personnel as the key to the whole program, and points out that although such units are expensive to operate, the costliness will prove worthwhile in terms of lives saved.

73. QUERIDO, A. *The Efficiency of Medical Care.* Leiden: Stenfert Kroese N.V., 1963.

An account of the many investigations carried out by a created Office for Public Health Care in Amsterdam for purposes of planning and development. Studies were undertaken in the areas of (a) the family physician, (b) prevention, (c) the hospital, (d) mental health, (e) geriatrics, (f) long-term illness and handicaps, and (g) the integrative approach. However, only those which specifically deal with evaluating the quality of care rendered (as opposed to cost analysis or availability) will be summarized below.

(a) Five practices were observed over a long period of time. Also, for each practice a five percent random sample of these patients (total 125 families) was visited and a routine physical was given to all family members. Psychological and social problems were assessed in terms of stress felt by the patient.

An inventory of what the physician did for a patient prior to hospital admission or before referral to a specialist was used as an index to the level of his activities. Two hundred ninety admissions and two hundred fifty referrals, both randomized from a given date, were reviewed by three physicians after admission and at the time of referral.

(b) The prenatal care of 212 perinatal deaths out of 8,590 deliveries over an eight-month period was examined by a physician who specialized in obstetrics. Twelve variables were taken into account. Further methodology is not defined, but it was determined that improvement of prenatal care might influence perinatal mortality only slightly.

To evaluate the effectiveness of the school health services in terms of abnormalities detected for the first time, screening done by four school physicians was observed and findings were analyzed.

A weight-coefficient was chosen as an indicator of nutritional condition. Number of kilograms per meter body length was calculated for a 10 percent sample of a year's school population. From each age group, two-and-a-half percent children were selected with the highest coefficient and two-and-a-half percent with the lowest. Data on the children's circumstances and conditions were gathered for each group. The chi square method was applied to test the derived data against chance probability. The weight-coefficient proved to be a sensitive index.

School absenteeism was also investigated as a possible indicator of health service. For each absenteeism in four schools during 38 weeks, a form was filled out and supplemented by a home visit. Frequency and duration of absenteeism, motivation for it, medical reason, and ten environmental circumstances were analyzed.

(c) Administrative reasons for length of stay in hospital were investigated by following every order given to a sample of patients. Ineffective days, without medical grounds, making no progress toward the purpose of the admission, were counted.

Frequency with which patients in an outpatient service followed advice was considered an index of "efficiency." Three months after a last visit, the patient was interviewed by a physician to determine reasons for his failure to follow medical advice. These reasons were then related to the outpatient unit which served the patient.

(d) Ex-pupils of a special school were interviewed 25 years after they left the school, and public and medical files were searched for information. They were assessed as to social adjustment and interhuman relations on a four-point scale. Since there was no control group, the figures derived cannot answer the question whether the services of the school were effective.

A country house was staffed by a psychiatrist, case worker, a chief supervisor, and eight group supervisors to give 24 selected children an accepting and emotionally healthy environment. The therapy proved useful over ambulatory care for certain kinds of impairments.

(e) To test the effectiveness of service to hospital patients that includes attention to their social and psychological relations as well as somatic problems, an inventory of psychosocial conditions was obtained on a random sample of patients. The concept of subjective distress was emphasized. A yes-no question form was filled out by the ward physician. Needs of the patients were assessed with respect to services received and what should be offered.

The psychosocial inquiry form was also used to answer whether patients who, after hospital admission for surgical treatment, were found to be cured, i.e., significantly more free from nonsomatic distress than patients found not to be cured.

The outcome of a group of posthospital patients who had had a clinical assessment was compared with that of patients who had been given the "integrative" assessment. A general ward physician made a prognosis in light of a clinical history and then a follow-up was done. Follow-up was also done on 1,630 who had had the psychosocial history. The factors investigated (demographic, presence of stress, follow-up assessment) were assumed to be independent of each other, but were considered related if the differences between actual results and expected results were larger than chance probability. Also, the accuracy of prognosis from the two approaches was tested against follow-up observations. This was analyzed diagramatically. It was shown that the type of distress had no specific influence on recovery. To test if the nature of distress had any influence, the factors causing distress were categorized and patients in one category were compared with the remainder. It was confirmed that presence of distress has a "decisive influence" on the chance of recovery, but the nature of it is immaterial.

In each of the studies the conclusions and possible implications are discussed, with tables presenting the findings.

74. RAE, J. W.; E. W. SMITH; and A. LENZER. Results of a rehabilitation program for geriatric patients in county hospitals. *J. Amer. Med. Assoc.* 180 (6):463–468, May 12, 1962.

This study attempts to test the effectiveness of rehabilitation programs set up for geriatric patients in three of Michigan's county institutions, each of which included physical restorative services, recreational activities and sheltered workshops. A fourth hospital was designated as the control. The study population consisted of 208 patients, with a median age of 80, who were given rehabilitation treatments for six months. Each individual was given an initial total medical evaluation and categorized into one of four categories descriptive of his or her ability to perform several activities of daily living with varying degrees of assistance from the personnel. Rehabilitation program effectiveness was judged both by the functional improvement and by the eligibility for discharge attained by termination of treatment. The experimental group exhibited greater strides both in functional improvement and discharge eligibility than did the controls. Substantial savings in public welfare funds also resulted.

75. SANAZARO, PAUL J.; and JOHN W. WILLIAMSON. End results of patient care: a provisional classification based on reports by internists. *Medical Care* 6(2):123–130, March–April, 1968.

(Author summary) A modification of the critical-incident technique was applied to a carefully selected group of internists [from 20 medical schools located in 14 states] engaged in the full-time private practice of medicine and holding volunteer faculty titles at medical schools. The end results contained in their written reports of patient care episodes were classified into twelve categories. The categories are defined as comprising two groups: patient end results and process outcomes. The frequency of mention of social, psychological, and physical functioning as end results suggests these were considered by the reporting physicians to be their appropriate concerns, along with purely medical outcomes. However, the limitations inherent in the source of the data preclude any generalizations.

The comprehensive description of categories of outcomes is proposed as a point of departure for developing specific criteria and techniques for validating current professional judgments of what constitutes effective performance by an interist. Further prospective empirical studies are required to determine whether the classification and its future modifications can provide an index for assessing patient care objectively and reliably.

76. SHAPIRO, SAM; JOSEPHINE J. WILLIAMS; ALONZO S. YERBY; PAUL M. DENSEN; and HENRY ROSNER. Patterns of medical use by the indigent aged under two systems of medical care. *Amer. J. Pub. Hlth.* 57(5):784–790, May, 1967.

During a year, 1963–1964, 13,000 public assistance recipients in New York City enrolled in HIP groups and 1,500 nursing home patients so enrolled were compared with OAA recipients not enrolled. Welfare records and HIP records provided information. This paper does not detail methodology, which can be found in a Final Report to the Health Research Council (New York City). It does summarize the findings on similarities and differences in patterns of use, mortality, and costs.

77. THOMPSON, JOHN D.; DON B. MARQUIS; ROBERT L. WOODWARD; and RICHARD C. YEOMANS. End-result measurements of the quality of obstetrical care in two U.S. Air Force hospitals. *Med. Care* 6(2):131–143, March, 1968.

A portion of this paper is devoted to a review of the problems of obstetrical end-result studies—variables, comparisons, availability and consistency of data, measurement factors—and specific characteristics of hospital perinatal studies, with reference to limitations, findings, and methods of previous obstetrical studies. The reported study was carried out in two U.S. Air Force hospitals, comparable in service and where most of the subjects received their prenatal care in the hospitals. Perinatal and submaturity rates were analyzed in relation to race, age, and parity of mother and to trimester in which prenatal care began. Different patterns of end results existed by race and parity, though no difference was found between the races in utilization. A special study was made of mothers in one of the two hospitals to identify factors contributing to high risk of unfavorable outcome.

IMPLEMENTATION AND EFFECTIVENESS OF UTILIZATION REVIEW

78. AMERICAN HOSPITAL ASSOCIATION. Guiding principles for hospital utilization review programs. *Hospitals* 40:75,76,131, March 16, 1966.

   This is a statement on hospital utilization review programs by the American Hospital Association which gives 13 suggestions for a review committee. The statements concern organizational points, general principles, responsibilities, composition and duties of the committee.

79. AMERICAN HOSPITAL ASSOCIATION. Guiding principles for utilization review programs for extended care facilities. *Hospitals* 40 (15 Part I):73,76, 68, August 1, 1966.

   A statement of twelve principles approved by the Board of Trustees of the American Hospital Association.

80. CRISTO, CARMEN. "Handbook: The Extended Care Facility and Utilization Review." In *The Extended Care Facility: A Handbook for the Medical Society*. Chicago: American Medical Association, 1967. pp. 17–48.

   A utilization review plan should include specifications in four general areas: organization and structure of the committee; responsibilities of the various parties; type of case to be reviewed and method of selection; forms, reports, procedures, meetings. The author interprets conditions of P.L. 89–97 as they relate to these four areas, giving detailed guidance for setting up a review plan. Copies of sample forms are included. The second part of this Handbook is an account of a pilot study of a regional utilization review project in Monroe County, New York, using a sample of six institutions which provide extended care facilities. Each institution randomly selected a given number of cases and completed a Nursing Evaluation Sheet and upper portion of the Extended Care Facility Case Review Form prior to arrival of the physician surveyors. Results were centrally collected and a meeting with the surveyors provided further information as pertinent. Problems were encountered such as defining levels of care and placing patients in proper facilities existing at the local level, and in the lag of recording in the medical chart. The author discusses these and indicates the time involved by professionals in this project.

81. HASSARD, HOWARD. Medical society review programs. *J. Amer. Med. Assoc.* 196(11):1004–1006, June 13, 1966.

   Prior to Medicare the California Medical Association (CMA) attempted to develop self-disciplinary mechanisms for the medical profession designed to assist the public in four key areas of medical care: (1) cost; (2) quality; (3) availability; and (4) scope of service. Hassard describes one portion of this effort—the CMA pioneer program "Guiding Principles for Physician-Hospital Relationships"—which endorses the concept of medical staff review committees to consider such procedures as applicant investigation, staff performance, and utilization. This program is in the process of being evaluated by medical staff survey committees comprised of independent CMA physician members; latest results show that 105 of the 174 staffs reviewed were approved. New efforts are being made to apply like principles to physicians in long-term care facilities. Since passage of Public Law 89-97, California has passed legislation to implement Title XIX, one provision of which calls for the establishment of a 16-member "Health Review and Program Council," a broadly defined review and planning group designed to spread the utilization concept to outpatient treatment. The claims review procedures of several California county societies are discussed, as well as the liability of the physician member of a medical society or hospital staff committee.

82. HOSPITAL UTILIZATION PROJECT. *Guide to Establishment and Functioning of a Medical Staff Utilization Committee.* [Pittsburgh]: Blue Cross of Western Pennsylvania, July, 1965.

This is a booklet developed by the Tenth Councilor District of the Pennsylvania Medical Society and the Hospital Council of Western Pennsylvania. The Guide sets forth the mechanics of establishing a Utilization Committee, the relationships necessary with other hospital committees, and four ways the administration can be of assistance to the committee. Specific advice on committee functioning is given concerning especially: review of charts, number of charts to be reviewed, classes of charts to be reviewed, review irrespective of payment, and committee activity independent of occupancy. Recommendations are made concerning follow-up, reports, and record-keeping. Two review forms are included in the appendix. (Also printed in *Utilization Review, A Handbook for the Medical Staff.* Chicago: American Medical Association, 1965.)

83. KLUTCH, MURRAY. Medical society review committees. *Inquiry* 2(2):70-76, September, 1965.

After briefly surveying the number and kind of society review committees across the country the author relates experience in three counties in California under the aegis of the State Medical Association. Review of claims forms was the mechanism adopted. Each county selected a list of diseases and formulated criteria for each. Only preliminary findings were available for reporting here. Future research/study plans and the expressed reasons for resistance from some of the county societies are presented.

84. KOLB, JONATHAN; and VICTOR W. SIDEL. Influence of utilization review on hospital length of stay. *J. Amer. Med. Assn.* 203(2):117-119, January, 1968.

At the Massachusetts General Hospital, the hypothesis that the utilization review mechanism is effective in altering lengths of stay for Medicare Part A beneficiaries was tested. Discharges for patients 65 and older for the third quarter of 1966 were compared with those of the third quarter of 1964, a pre-Medicare control group. The results are presented with various possible interpretations. A significantly higher proportion of Medicare patients was discharged in 18 to 21 days, while the under-14-day period showed lower for the Medicare group and the over-25-day period higher. The authors believe that pre-Medicare stays were probably too short because of financial constraints, and that arbitrary limitation is a more effective device but that utilization review may be more selective in reducing length of stay.

85. LETOURNEAU, CHARLES. A look at utilization of medical and hospital services. *Hospital Manag.* 94:47–50, September, 1962.

This article disputes the statement that the physicians and hospitals are guilty of gross waste of hospitalization in unnecessary admissions or long hospital stays. The author states the functions of the utilization committee to allow physicians fair treatment in getting patients into the hospital, to review long-stay patients, and to check use of services. He cautions against a too powerful position for the committee.

86. LONDON, MORRIS. Medical staff utilization committees. *Inquiry* 2(2):77–95, September, 1965.

A discussion of goals, problems, and organization of utilization committees in general and a current and historic appraisal of the HUP program of western Pennsylvania in particular. The formulation of criteria for 50 diagnoses by panels of academic and practicing physicians is discussed. Also a special study wherein seven hospital utilization committees reviewed the same two diagnoses using the criteria lists is described. Included with the article are reprints of the work sheets for two conditions along with the criteria used, and copies of the abstract sheets and monthly reports to the hospitals, by disease category.

87. MCCLENAHAN, EVERETT. Hospital utilization reviews. *J. Amer. Med. Assoc.* 196(11):99–104, June 13, 1966.

The author points out the differences between utilization committees pre-Medicare and post-Medicare. He then prescribes five principles of a "proper utilization committee," and outlines those features a record librarian, as well as a committee, must look for. The structure and function of four types of committees are described—that for a large hospital, medium-sized hospital, a small hospital, and a specialty hospital. Using data from the Hospital Utilization Project in Pittsburgh, the author describes an example of an interdepartmental comparison concerned with OR use, a profile of a physician by using a cholecystectomy case, and an interhospital study of deliveries by three obstetricians in each of two hospitals.

88. MCCLENAHAN, J. EVERETT. "Applying the Results of Utilization Measurement." In *National Conference on Utilization*. Chicago: March 2–8, 1962, Report Series #2. Amer. Hospital Assoc., 1962.

In the face of increased medical costs and a crisis in financing of voluntary medical care, the Tenth Councilor District Program in Western Pennsylvania was set up to insure high-quality care at reasonable costs in a system adaptive to group payment or insurance principles. The Program consists of five committees one of which is a Utilization Committee. This is discussed in terms of fact-finding, educational responsibilities, membership, relationship to hospital, meeting frequency, and pertinent issues for discussion. The author makes specific suggestions for the number of charts to be reviewed, describes the mechanism of a claims review committee in detail, delineates benefits and pitfalls of utilization review, and lists ingredients of an effective committee.

BIBLIOGRAPHY

89. SHARPE, GEORGE. A community-wide approach to utilization review. *Chronic Illness Newsletter* 18(6):2–5, December, 1967.

> In Montgomery County, Maryland, a Community Coordinating Committee was set up under the auspices of the Medical Society to deal with integrating extended care services into various levels of medical care. A community-based utilization plan to review stays of extended duration was supported by Public Health Service. From the Society membership, two-physician teams are drawn and rotated among the 10 ECF institutions participating. This paper describes the function of the review team, the review process, results of the developing program, and some of the problems encountered.

90. SIGMOND, ROBERT M. "Controlling Hospital Use Through Medical Staff Utilization Committees." In *Where is Hospital Use Headed? Fifth Annual Symposium on Hospital Affairs, Proceedings.* Chicago: University of Chicago, 1962, pp. 73–80.

> Medical and hospital leaders in Western Pennsylvania have developed a program to control inpatient utilization through reduction of length of stay and increase in occupancy rate. The program stresses that it is the physician, not the patient, who utilizes hospital services, and thus the individual utilization committee is concerned with educating medical staffs about their impact on utilization rates. Questionnaires were sent in 1960 and 1961 to 38 hospitals in the Tenth Councilor District of the Pennsylvania Medical Society to determine how the utilization committees have been functioning during their first two years. Descriptions are included of committee size, frequency of meetings, types of charts reviewed, and type of action on "questionable" utilization. The hospitals reported many changes and improvements in hospital procedures which resulted from utilization review. The author discusses several common misconceptions of utilization committees, makes suggestions for effective utilization committees, and analyzes cetain weaknesses.

91. SMITH, PAUL R. Case review mechanisms. *Inquiry* 2(2):64–69, September, 1965.

> Philadelphia Blue Cross has a four-step plan: (a) a group is notified of every admission; (b) follow-up is done at the company's discretion; (c) employee patient completes a questionnaire about his stay; a nurse reviews records of selected cases and records pertinent information on the questionnaire form; a physician reconstructs the case; (d) a meeting is held with the utilization committee. The cost of the program per case is indicated.

STANDARDS

92. THE AMERICAN COLLEGE OF OBSTETRICIANS AND GYNECOLOGISTS. *Manual of Standards of Obstetric-Gynecologic Practice.* Chicago: The College, 1965, 120 pp.

    These standards cover physical facilities and equipment, obstetrical patient care, gynecological practice, including proper consultation, medical records and statistics, and samples of 19 patient and reporting forms.

93. AMERICAN COLLEGE OF SURGEONS, COMMITTEE ON TRAUMA. Standards for emergency ambulance services. *Bull. Amer. Coll. of Surg.* 52(3):131-132, May-June, 1967.

    Set up by the Committee on Trauma of the American College of Surgeons Board of Regents in 1967, these standards cover: organization and operation; personnel; vehicles; equipment; communications.

94. CASHMAN, JOHN W.; and BEVERLEE A. MYERS. Medicare: standards of service in a new program—licensure, certification, accreditation. *Amer. J. Pub. Hlth.* 57(7):1107-1117, July, 1967.

    This is a description to date of achievements in defining and applying standards for the Medicare program, and how standards differ from licensure and accreditation. The authors review the public, professional, and political influences which affect such differences. They describe the problems encountered in setting standards especially for home health agencies, extended care facilities, and independent laboratories; the current weaknesses; and relationships between the federal program and local agencies. Experience with application of standards is presented for hospitals only, since that for other types of facilities was as yet too limited. Other problems such as the "quality-availability" dichotomy, and widely varying interpretations of the qualitative terms in which the standards were stated, are discussed. There is a look into future prospects and what remains to be done.

95. COMMISSION ON CANCER. Manual for Cancer Programs. Chicago: American College of Surgeons [1965].

    Contains procedures and requisites for approval, basic standards, and samples of cancer registry report forms.

96. GRYNBAUM, BRUCE B.; and ELIZABETH SPEARE. Quality control in an urban amputee program. *Amer. J. Pub. Hlth.* 56(8):1199-1204, August, 1966.

    The paper contains excerpts from Guide for the Establishment of Amputee Centers in New York City. Progress achieved in applying the standards is outlined.

97. RICE, R. GERALD (Michigan Crippled Children Commission). "Standards of Care for Public Health Programs for Mothers and Children." In *Institute on the Development of Community Health Services for Children with Congenital Anomalies.* Ann Arbor: University of Michigan School of Public Health, 1964, pp. 74-87.

    (Author summary) An overview of standards of care as seen by an administrator has been presented. Standards have been discussed from

BIBLIOGRAPHY

the point of view of definition and purpose, of basic essentials, of types, of origin, and of blocks to their utilization. The knowledge needed to improve quality of care is available; all administrators require is the courage to use it.

98. TRUSSELL, RAY E. Proprietary nursing home standards in New York City. *Amer. J. Pub. Hlth.* 56(8):1261–1270, August, 1966.

A committee of approximately 80 persons, representing government agencies, voluntary and proprietary institutions, and various experts, assisted the Department of Hospitals in updating a code which governs licensure and supervision of proprietary nursing homes. This paper quotes highlights of the code, especially in regard to patient care and rights. The author recounts some of the results of the code in force.

EVALUATION IN NURSING

99. GORHAM, WILLIAM A. Methods for measuring staff nursing performance. *Nurs. Res.* 12(1):4–11, Winter, 1963.

> In another paper, nursing behaviors contributing to patient care and improvement were identified. The measurements developed therefrom were to identify personnel strengths and weaknesses in specific performance areas, and the head nurse was to function as an on-the-job observer and reporter. A Profile Checklist compared a staff nurse's performance in one of five behavioral categories against her performance in the other four. A Graphic Rating judges the nurse against others in each of the five areas plus an overall performance rating. A Forced Profile is very much like the Checklist and distributes 100 points among the five areas. In the Preference Checklist the observer checks the statement in a pair which best describes the nurse's typical performance. In the Observation Record the observer notes specific incidents of effective or ineffective performance. The Observation Checklist groups 100 items into the 5 areas from which the observer chooses each day those behaviors she observed about each nurse that day. These six instruments were tried out over a three-week period in two District of Columbia hospitals with similar nurse staffing patterns, though one was with a school program. All measures were evaluated in terms of relevance, reliability, rater errors, objectivity, predictability, and acceptability, and the author discusses each of these criteria.

100. PHANEUF, MARIA C. Analysis of a nursing audit. *Nurs. Outlook* 16(1): 57–60, January, 1968.

> The details of the methodology of this Audit are to be found in earlier articles in *Nursing Outlook*, May 1964 and June 1966. This paper presents results of the audit when applied to records of 500 patients in 20 community nursing service agencies. Seven categories of nursing functions and 50 derived components were used as the standard. Tables are presented for each of the seven functions for this randomized sample, with a discussion of the weaknesses revealed by the low scores.

101. REITER, FRANCES; and MARGUERITE E. KAKOSH. *Quality of Nursing Care: A Report of a Field-Study To Establish Criteria—1950–1954.* New York: Graduate School of Nursing, New York Medical College, 1964, 138 pp.

> "A recently published report of a four-year field study (1950–1954) done to establish criteria for the appraisal of nursing care. Answers were sought to the following questions: (1) What constitutes quality in nursing care? (2) What are the differences in the quality of nursing approaches, activities, understandings, and skills in relation to the effectiveness of nursing care that patients receive? (3) Can the components of nursing care be identified and how can they be described in an instrument or guide for purposes of qualitative appraisal? The study consisted of: (1) the collection and analysis of descriptions of nursing care; (2) categorization of types of nursing care; (3) development, use and revision of observation guide; and (4) development of a seminar in 'listening skills.' The descriptions of nursing care were

used to identify, define, and examine segments of nursing care. The final categories of nursing care were: Type I, Professional; Type II, Technical; and Type III, Elementary. Nurses were able to sense differences in the quality of nursing care more reliably by recognition than by recall. Therefore, the Observation Guide contains questions which focus the observers' attention on the quality of direct nursing care. Nurse operations were clustered around four major nursing operations: ministration, observation, communication, and teaching. Behavioral criteria were identified in each of the nursing operations for each of the three types of nursing care. Most of the care observed could be assigned to Types II and III. There were few instances of Type I observed in the actual hospital setting" (abstract from *Nursing Research* Vol. 13).

102. ROSEN, ALBERT; and GERTRUDE E. ABRAHAM. Evaluation of a procedure for assessing the performance of staff nurses. *Nurs. Res.* 12(2):78–82, Spring, 1963.

This study (at a VA Hospital) is based on the critical incident technique and a Graphic Rating Form. The latter was developed by the American Institute for Research, and a revision of it used for this study was called the Nursing Performance Description Form, consisting of 50 items. This form, about nine staff nurses, was completed by staff nurses, supervisory nurses and medical residents. In addition, questionnaire information about the study nurses was added to a routine Proficiency Report. Also, the supervisory nurses filled out six Global Evaluation Forms for the total group of staff nurses. After repeat rating of the same staff nurses on the NPDF form, interrater agreement and consistency of each rater for the total score as well as for each item, were calculated. Validity of the NPDF items was tested against total scores. By computing correlation coefficients, interrelationships between the NPDF and Global Ratings and the NPDF and Proficiency Report were analyzed. Further, ratings among the three groups of raters were compared by analysis of variance. The NPDF total score proved valid but no better than the Proficiency Report or the Global Evaluation Form, both of which are simpler to use.

DRUG THERAPY AUDIT

103. MULLER, CHARLOTTE. Medical review of prescribing. *J. Chron. Dis.* 18 (7):689–696, July, 1965.

> Drug therapy practices in two New York City institutions (one, both inpatient and outpatient, the other, only outpatient) were studied by two physician reviewers, with a third to consult on some of the outpatient cases. Coded PAS forms for inpatients were used for initial screening of "acceptable" or "questionable" practices by one judge. Retabulation of criticized drugs was made after chart review, and the results were compared with judgments of a second reviewer who knew the first reviewer's opinions. For outpatients, similar coding and screening was done plus an evaluation of quantity prescribed and dispensed. In this phase, a testing of agreement between two reviewers was done through a judgment by Reviewer II without his knowledge of the first results. Further, results of a third judge were then obtained, and finally, Reviewer II consulted the patient charts. It was concluded that drug therapy screening without chart review is of little value. Tabulated results of drugs criticized, and further implications of the findings are presented.

104. MYERS, ROBERT S.; VERGIL N. SLEE; and RICHARD P. AMENT. Antibiotic study shows need for therapy audit in hospitals. *Bull. Amer. Coll. Surg.* 48(2):61–63, March–April, 1963.

> As recorded by PAS, discharges exclusive of births during January of 1959 and 1961 were examined for antibiotic use. While the percentage of patients given antibiotics went down (30 percent in 1961), use of antibiograms increased. Study of a random sample of 1961 discharges revealed that less than one-fourth had infections and only 60 percent of those received antibiotics. From another study of PAS data, a conservative figure of 12 percent was derived for patients needing antibiotics. The authors discuss frequency of antibiograms, misuse of antibiotics as prophylaxis, and how "therapy audit" may be applied.